Sankara Nethralaya's

Atlas of Uveitis and Scleritis

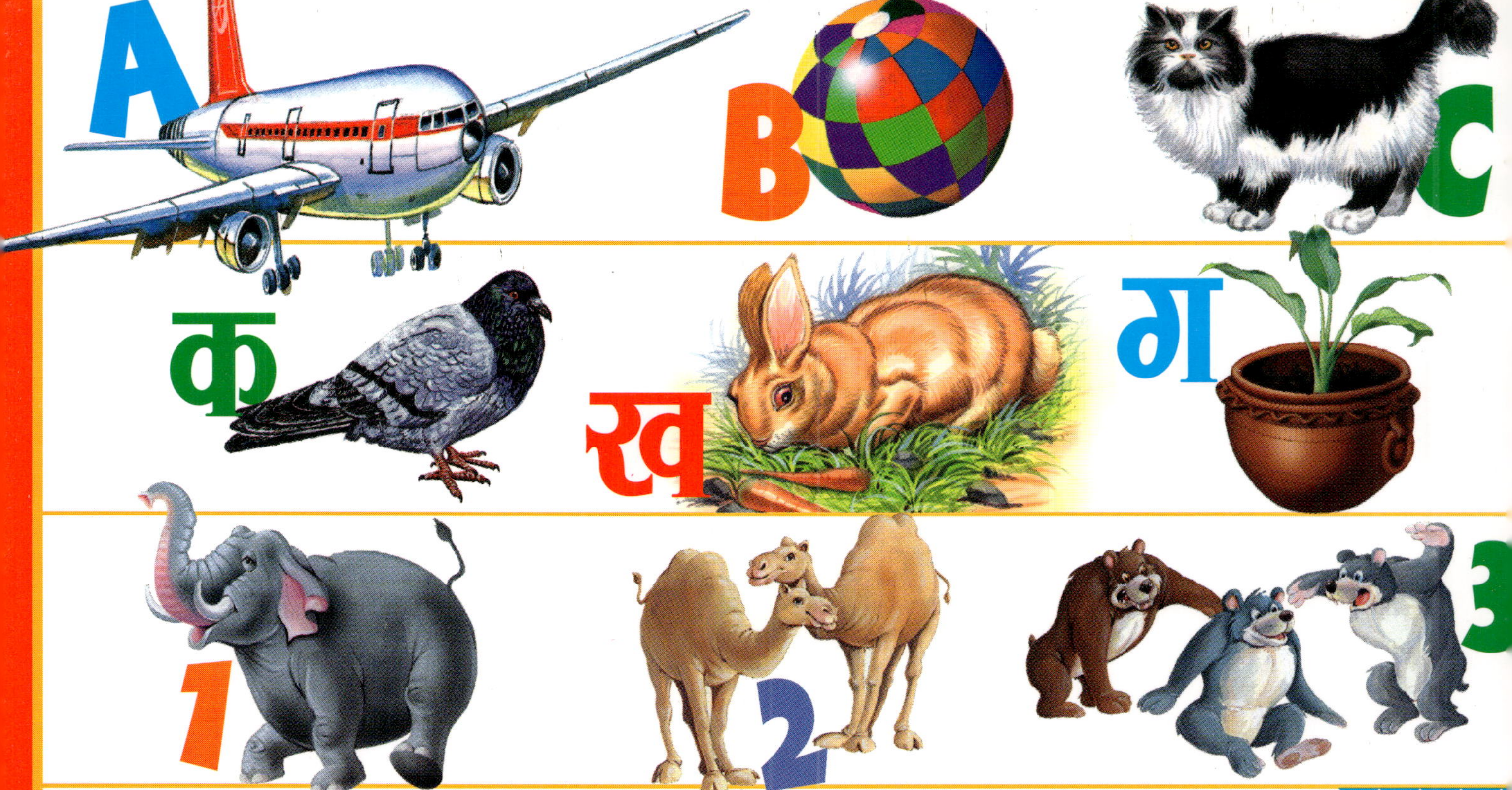
A
B
C
क
ख
ग
1
2
3

ALL IN ONE

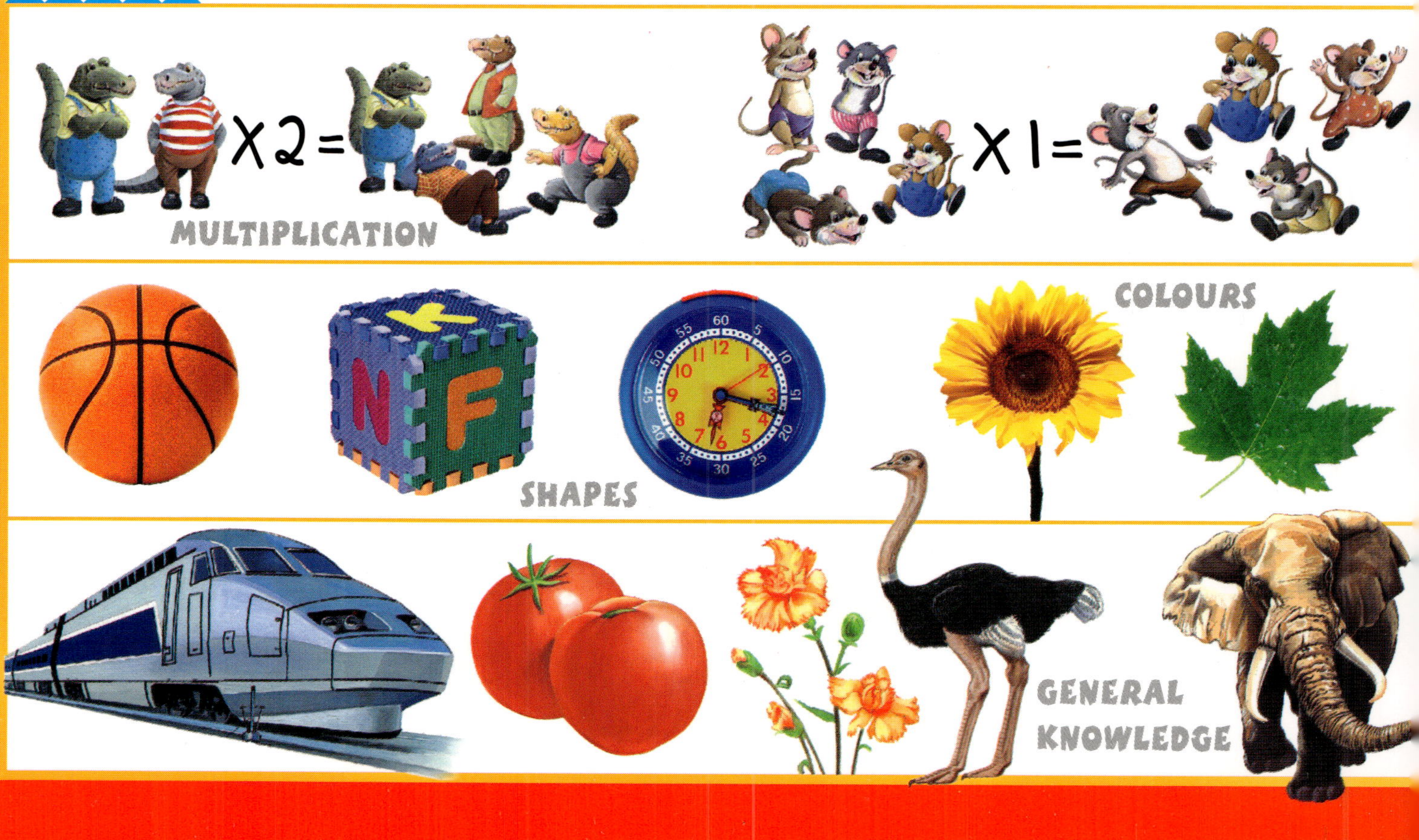
X 2 =
X 1 =
MULTIPLICATION
SHAPES
COLOURS
GENERAL KNOWLEDGE

Sankara Nethralaya's
Atlas of
Uveitis and Scleritis

Sudha K Ganesh
Mamta Agarwal
Amala E George
Jyotirmoy Biswas
Department of Uvea
Sankara Nethralaya, 18 College Road, Chennai

Taylor & Francis
Taylor & Francis Group
LONDON AND NEW YORK
A MARTIN DUNITZ BOOK

First published in India in 2005 by Jaypee Brothers Medical Publishers (P) Ltd, New Delhi, India.
First published by Taylor & Francis Medical Books, a member of the T&F-Informa Group plc in 2005. Exclusively distribut worldwide (excluding the Indian Subcontinent) by Taylor & Francis Medical Books, a member of the T&F-Informa Group plc

Tel.: +44 (0) 20 7017 6000
Fax.: +44 (0) 20 7017 6699
E-mail: info@dunitz.co.uk
Website: http://www.dunitz.co.uk

A CIP record for this book is available from the British Library.

ISBN 1 84184 550 7

Distributed in North and South America by

Taylor & Francis
2000 NW Corporate Blvd
Boca Raton, FL 33431, USA

Within Continental USA
Tel.: 800 272 7737; Fax.: 800 374 3401
Outside Continental USA
Tel.: 561 994 0555; Fax.: 561 361 6018
E-mail: orders@crcpress.com

Distributed in the rest of the world (excluding the Indian Subcontinent) by
Thomson Publishing Services
Cheriton House
North Way
Andover, Hampshire SP10 5BE, UK
Tel.: +44 (0)1264 332424
E-mail: salesorder.tandf@thomsonpublishingservices.co.uk

FOREWORD

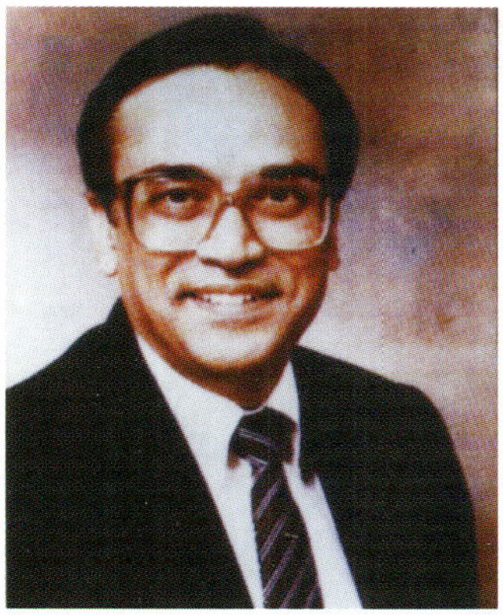

Several uveitic entities are recognized based on their clinical features and/or pathogenesis; such entities include Toxoplasma retinochoroiditis, Pars planitis, Serpiginous choroiditis and several others. In many instances however, determining exactly what initiated the process of uveitis has been a challenge, particularly when the trigger is an infectious agent. The detection process is complicated by the diverse clinical manifestations of uveitis that are induced by the infectious agent, by the unavailability of infected tissue for examination and by the lack of specific and sensitive diagnostic tests. For example, *Mycobacterium tuberculosis* can present with an anterior or posterior uveitis, with or without granulomas. Moreover this agent can induce a hypersensitivity reaction with clinical features of retinal vasculitis, iridocyclitis or multifocal choroiditis or with features suggestive of Serpiginous choroiditis. In such a clinical spectrum, *Mycobacterium tuberculosis* can be isolated from the granulomatous lesions, but such samples rarely become available. In hypersensitivity reactions such as retinal vasculitis, the infectious organisms appear to be absent from the retina, yet some patients respond positively to antituberculous agents suggesting that mycobacterium does indeed have a role in this entity. Sputum analysis and chest X-ray findings may not help pinpoint the diagnosis in these patients.

In recent years, molecular diagnostic procedures have detected infectious agents in some cases wherein organisms could not be cultured or detected by other microbiological procedures. Among the various molecular procedures used, the analysis of intraocular fluid by polymerase chain reaction (PCR) in uveitis has shown great promise in detecting traces of an infectious agent in the form of a microbial specific DNA sequence. This procedure has been successfully used by several laboratories including laboratory of Sankara Nethralaya to detect bacteria, viruses and protozoa in intraocular inflammation.

Based on well documented clinical findings, laboratory investigations including PCR analysis, the authors of this well illustrated atlas provide succinctly main clinical diagnostic features and management of various uveitic entities. The authors profusely illustrate clinical examples of both anterior and posterior uveitis and scleral inflammation seen in their practice over a decade. This atlas should be valuable to ophthalmologists in clinical practice and to postgraduate students who are in the process of acquiring knowledge in the field of uveitis, a leading cause of blindness in the developing world.

Narsing A Rao MD
Los Angeles, California
USA

PREFACE

Uveitis is an emerging subspeciality of ophthalmology that presents with a constellation of clinical findings. Accurate diagnosis of uveitis and successful treatment of these patients remain a challenge. The field of uveitis has been revolutionized over the past 50 years. Our understanding of ocular inflammatory diseases has progressed rapidly and we can accurately diagnose and treat these diseases. Basic science and research in immunology has led to new therapeutic approaches to the patient with uveitis and scleritis. This atlas gives the reader a concise overview of the clinical manifestations, investigations, diagnosis and management of uveitis and scleritis. We emphasize on careful clinical assessment and accurate diagnosis. This book is not intended to be a textbook but a practical guide to the diagnosis, in obtaining appropriate investigations and management. The uvea department has a team of four consultants and we examine about a thousand new cases of uveitis every year. The emphasis on maintaining good clinical record with digital archiving was an excellent source for selecting pictures for this atlas. All cases included were patients seen at Sankara Nethralaya, Chennai.

Authors

ACKNOWLEDGEMENTS

Dr SS Badrinath has been the driving force behind this atlas. Without his encouragement, this book would not have come into existence. We are deeply indebted to him for his active support.

We are very grateful to Mr SP Govindarajan, Mr S Jayaraman, Mr Anand and Ms Lakshmi (Nursing Staff) in photography department at Sankara Nethralaya. Special thanks to Dr Rajesh Fogla and Dr Mani Baskaran for their help in taking digital slit lamp photographs of the anterior segment.

We would like to give our special thanks to Mr V Murali, Mr Mohan and Mr Elango in our multimedia department who helped us in scanning the images. We also extend our sincere thanks to our corresponding secretaries. We also acknowledge the efforts of Jaypee Brothers Medical Publishers (P) Ltd for their technical assistance, printing and publishing this atlas on time. In particular, we like to thank Shri J P Vij, Chairman and Managing Director of Jaypee Brothers and Mr R Jayanandan, author Co-ordinator of Chennai branch.

Finally, we thank all our patients for trusting us and allowing us to participate in the management of their ocular problems.

CONTENTS

Section 1: Anterior Uveitis

Section 2: Intermediate Uveitis

Section 3: Posterior Uveitis

Section 4: Panuveitis

Section 5: Infectious Uveitis

Section 6: Systemic Diseases associated with Uveitis

Section 7: Complications of Uveitis

Section 8: Investigations in Uveitis

Section 9: Masquerade Syndrome

Section 10: Acquired Immunodeficiency Syndrome (AIDS)

Section 11: Scleritis

Section 1
Anterior Uveitis

CHAPTER ONE

Idiopathic Anterior Uveitis

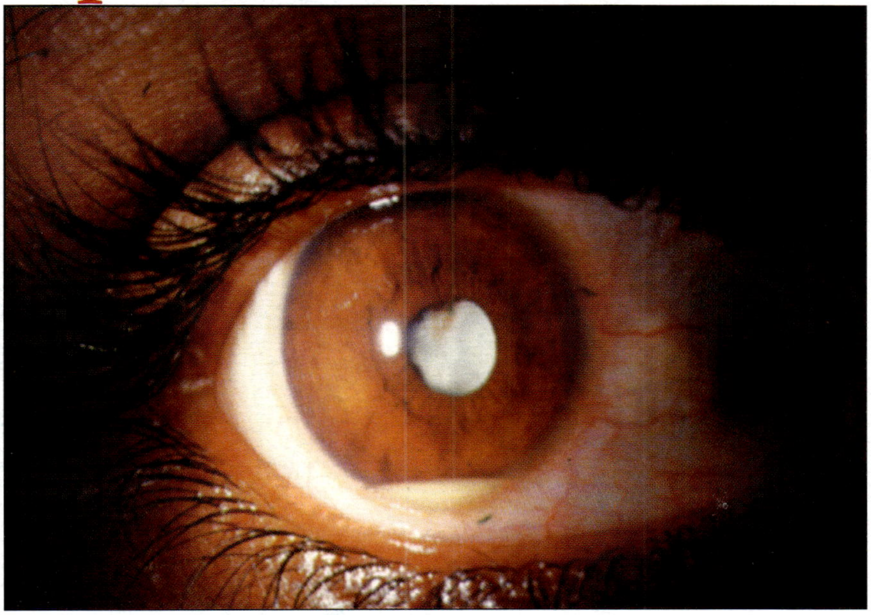

Inflammation of the iris and ciliary body is called anterior uveitis. It can be nongranulomatous or granulomatous.

Idiopathic nongranulomatous anterior uveitis is the most common type of anterior uveitis which is known to be associated with the human leukocyte antigen (HLA) B27 in 50-60 percent of patients. It is characterized by male predominance and may be associated with seronegative arthritic syndromes such as ankylosing spondylitis, Reiter syndrome, psoriatic arthritis, and inflammatory bowel disease.

Ocular Features

Symptoms

Pain, redness, photophobia, decreased vision.

Signs

Acute

- Circumcorneal congestion
- Fine keratic precipitates
- Aqueous flare and cells (graded according to severity)
- Hypopyon
- Posterior synechiae
- Iris bombé

Chronic

- Old pigmented keratic precipitates
- Broken posterior synechiae
- Seclusio and occlusio pupillae
- Posterior subcapsular cataract

Investigations

- Complete blood count
- Rheumatoid factor, antinuclear antibody
- Human leucocyte antigen (HLA-B27)

Treatment

- Topical steroids: Prednisolone acetate, Betamethasone, Dexamethasone. In acute cases, topical steroids can be used every hourly and gradually tapered.
- Cycloplegic agents: Atropine, Homatropine, Cyclopentolate
- In severe cases, periocular/ systemic steroids can be used.

REFERENCES

1. Biswas J, Narain S, Das D, Ganesh SK . Pattern of uveitis in a referral uveitis clinic in India. Int Ophthalmol. 1996-97;20:223-8.
2. Martin TM, Smith JR, Rosenbaum JT. Anterior uveitis: Current concepts of pathogenesis and interactions with the spondyloarthropathies. Curr Opin Rheumatol. 2002;14:337-41.

Clinical Features of Nongranulomatous Anterior Uveitis

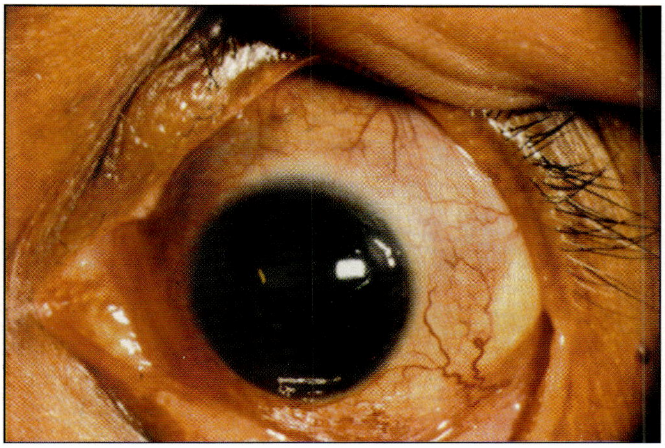

Fig. 1.1: Slit lamp photograph showing circumcorneal congestion in a case of acute anterior uveitis

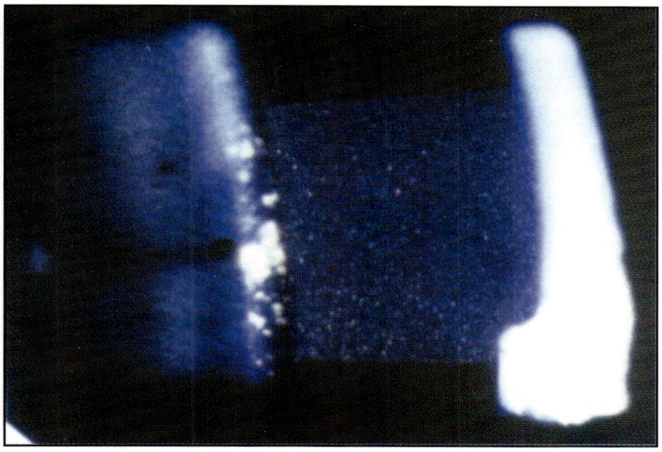

Fig. 1.2: Anterior chamber slit beam photograph showing intense flare due to breakdown of blood aqueous barrier

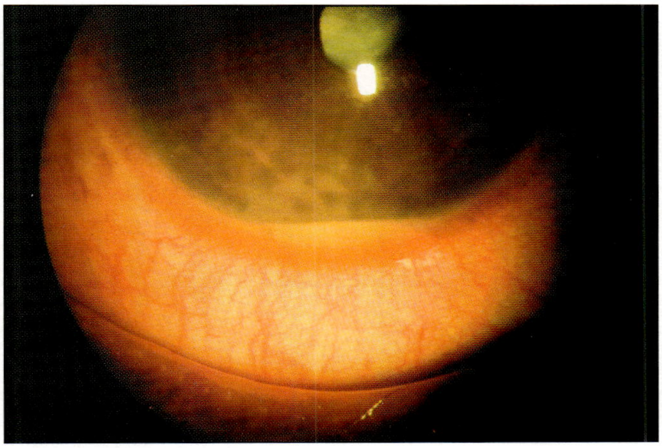

Fig. 1.3: Hypopyon in an HLA B27 positive patient with ankylosing spondylitis

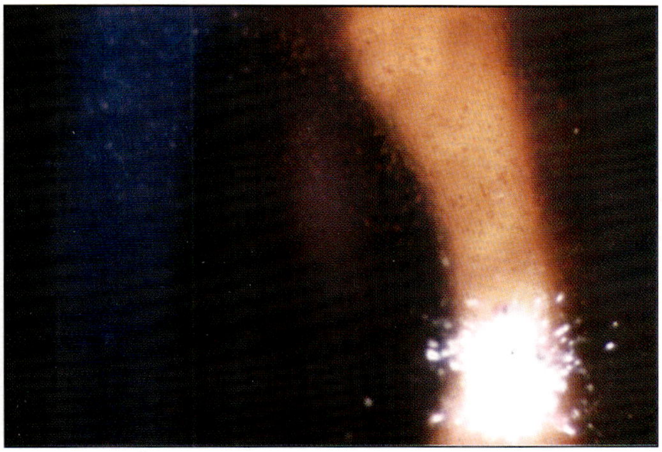

Fig. 1.4: Slit beam photograph showing small to medium sized keratic precipitates

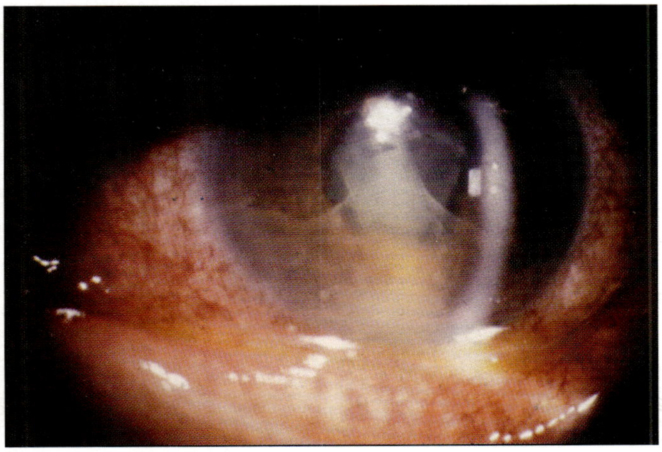

Fig. 1.5: Slit lamp examination of anterior chamber showing circumcorneal congestion, fine keratic precipitates , aqueous flare, cells and severe fibrinous reaction in anterior chamber

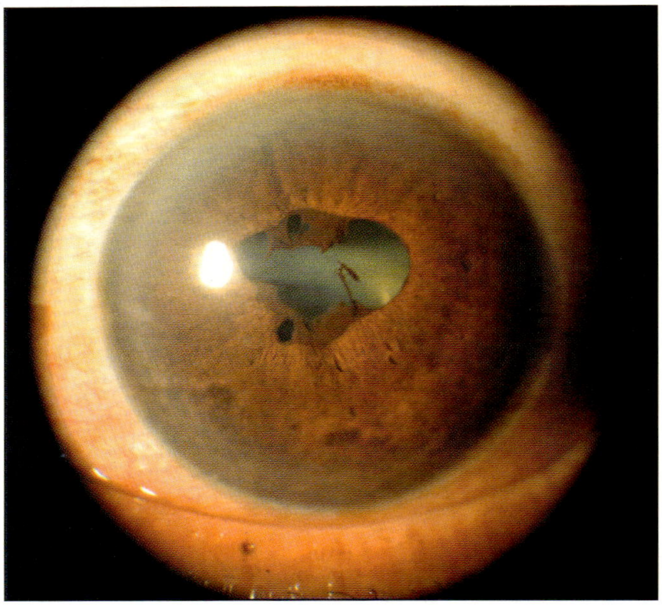

Fig. 1.6: Posterior synechiae following attacks of recurrent anterior uveitis

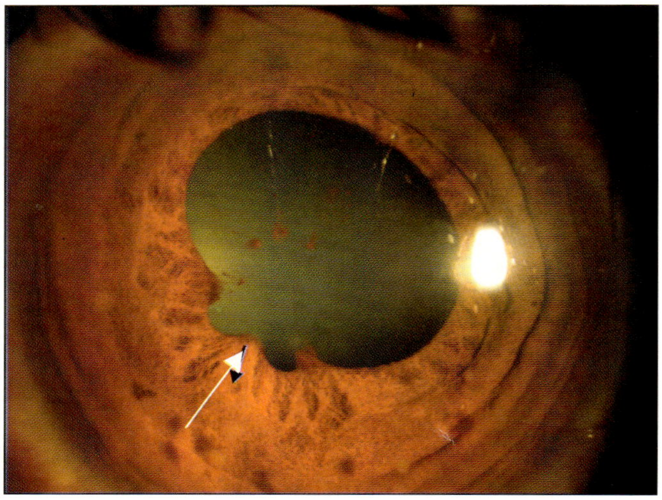

Fig. 1.7: Slit lamp photograph showing circumcorneal congestion, iris nodules and posterior synechiae (arrow)

Systemic Associations of Idiopathic Anterior Uveitis

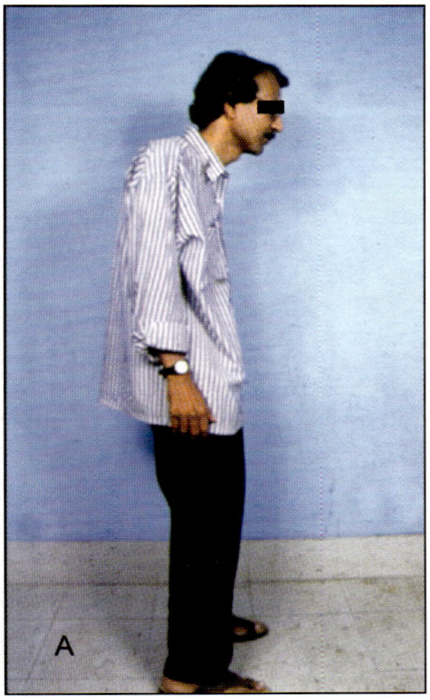

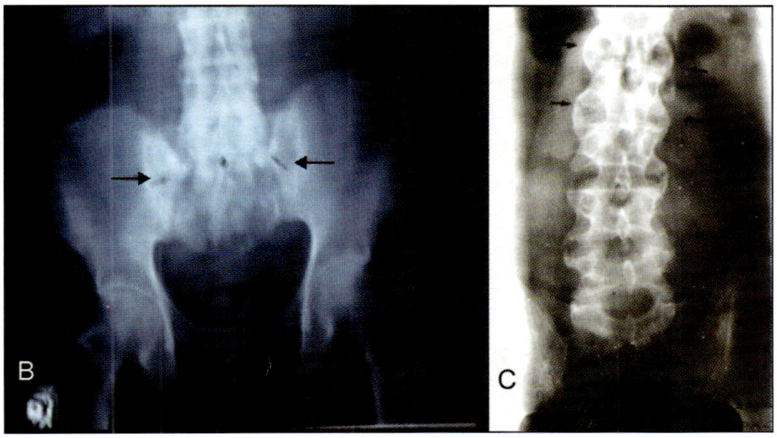

Figs 1.8A to C
A. A 40-year-old man suffering from ankylosing spondylitis
B. X-ray hip showed sclerosis of sacroiliac joints (arrows)
C. X-ray spine showed complete spinal fusion, i.e. bamboo spine

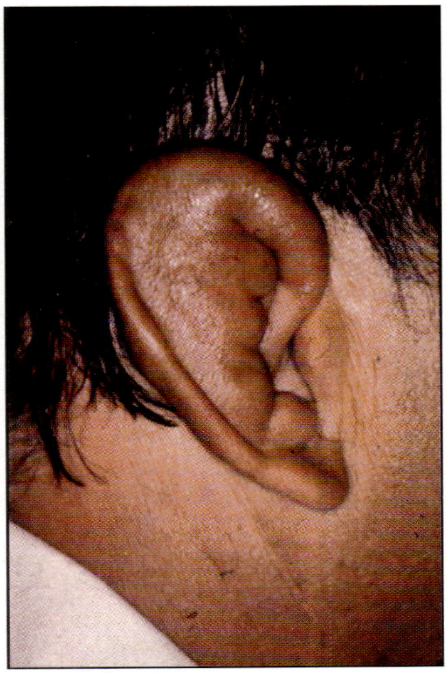

Fig. 1.9: Active chondritis involving the external ear in a patient with relapsing polychondritis who also developed recurrent attacks of anterior uveitis

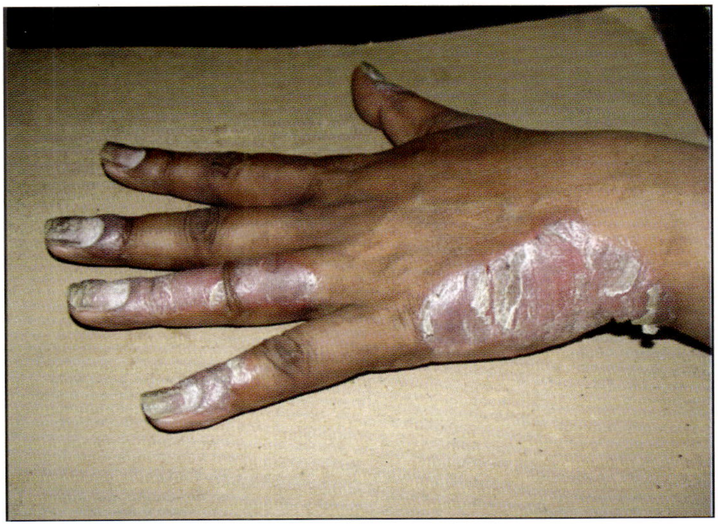

Fig. 1.10: External photograph of a patient with psoriasis showing exfoliative skin lesions with silvery scales, onycholysis, pitting and nail discoloration along with swelling of distal interphalangeal joints (sausage digits).

CHAPTER TWO

Granulomatous Anterior Uveitis

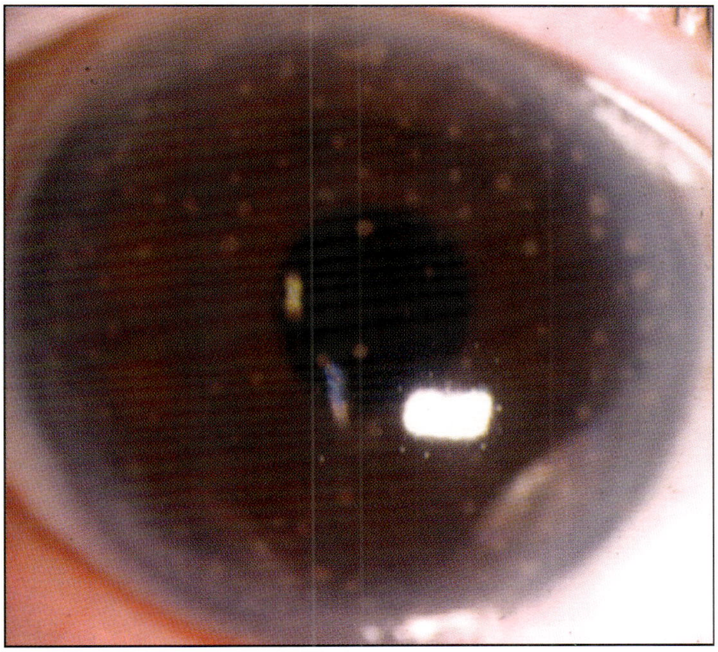

Granulomatous anterior uveitis is a chronic subclinical inflammation of the iris and ciliary body. It may be due to an idiopathic reaction or from the host's immune response to a systemic infectious process such as syphilis, tuberculosis, Hansen's disease or local reactivation of herpetic viral infection or sarcoidosis. It is usually bilateral, involve all parts of the eye and can be part of a systemic disease process or an ocular syndrome.

Ocular Features

Symptoms

Decreased vision, dull aching eye, pain, photophobia.

Signs

External

- Herpetic uveitis—Cutaneous vesicles in the distribution of the ophthalmic branch of the fifth cranial nerve
- Hansen's disease—Madarosis, leonine facies

Ocular

- No circumcorneal congestion
- Large (mutton-fat) keratic precipitates
- Aqueous flare and cells
- Koeppe nodules, Busacca's nodules
- Sectoral iris atrophy in herpetic uveitis
- Generalized iris atrophy in Hansen's disease
- Raised intraocular pressure especially in herpetic uveitis
- Inflammatory nodules in the angle

Investigations

- Complete blood count
- Erythrocyte sedimentation rate
- Mantoux test
- Serum angiotensin converting enzyme
- Fluorescent treponemal antibody absorption test (FTA-ABS)
- Venereal Disease Research Laboratory Test (VDRL)
- Rapid Plasma Reagin (RPR)
- Chest X-ray

Treatment

- Topical steroids: Prednisolone acetate, Betamethasone, Dexamethasone
- Cycloplegic agents: Atropine, Homatropine, Cyclopentolate
- Treatment of specific diseases (Tuberculosis, syphilis, sarcoidosis, Hansen's disease)
- In case of noninfectious posterior segment involvement, systemic steroids / immunosuppressive agents are required.

REFERENCES

1. Kristeva M, Biswas J, Pararajasegaram G, Sevanian A and Rao NA: 'Histochemical analysis of experimental granulomatous uveitis'. Ophthalmic Research. 1991; 23:73-78.
2. Nussenblatt RB, Whitcup SM, Palestine AG: Uveitis: Fundamentals and Clinical Practice. 2nd edn. Mosby-Year Book; 1996.
3. Rao NA, Cousins S, Forster D: Intraocular Inflammation and Uveitis: Basic and Clinical Science Course 2002.

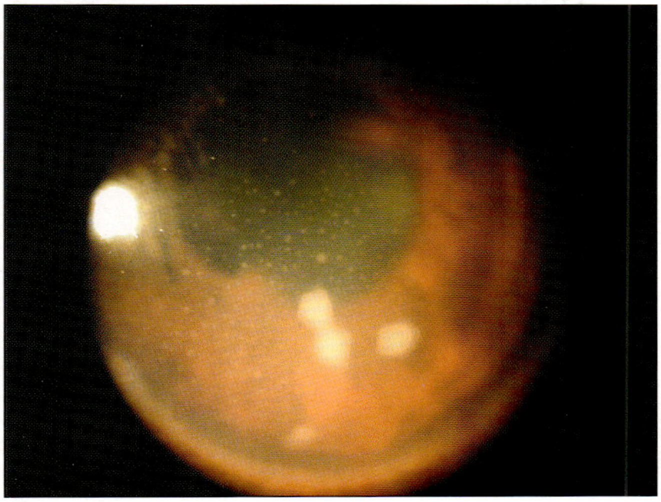

Fig. 2.1: Multiple mutton-fat keratic precipitates in a patient with sarcoidosis

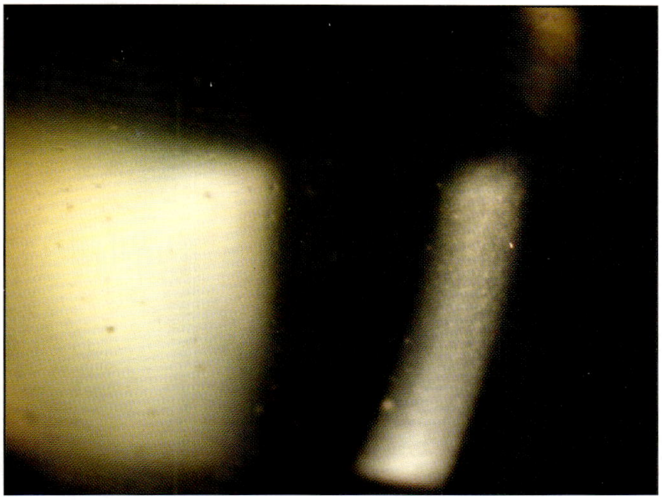

Fig. 2.2: Slit lamp photograph shows large, round, translucent keratic precipitates in a patient with Hansen's disease

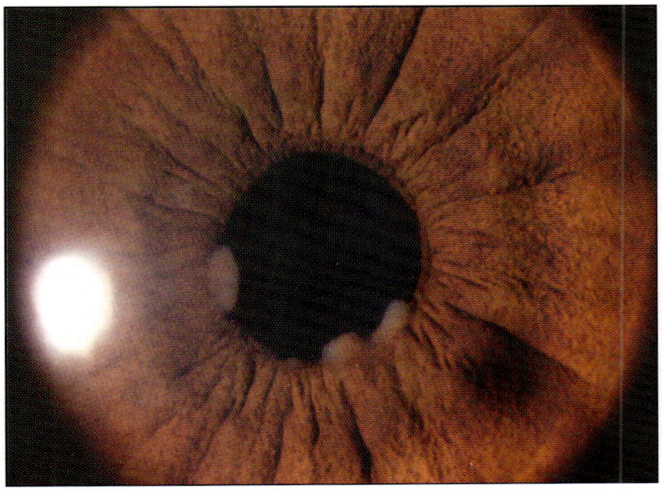

Fig. 2.3: Koeppes nodules at the pupillary border in a case of sarcoidosis

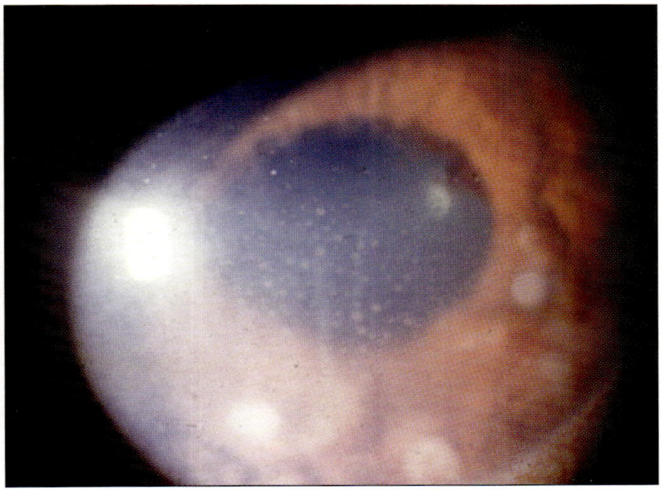

Fig. 2.4: Slit lamp photograph showing large iris nodules (Busacca nodules) and keratic precipitates in a patient with pulmonary tuberculosis

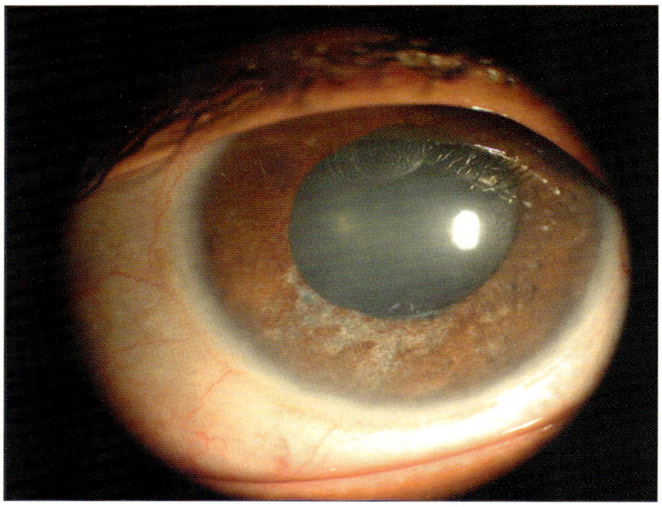

Fig. 2.5: Slit lamp photograph showing sectoral iris atrophy in a patient with herpetic anterior uveitis

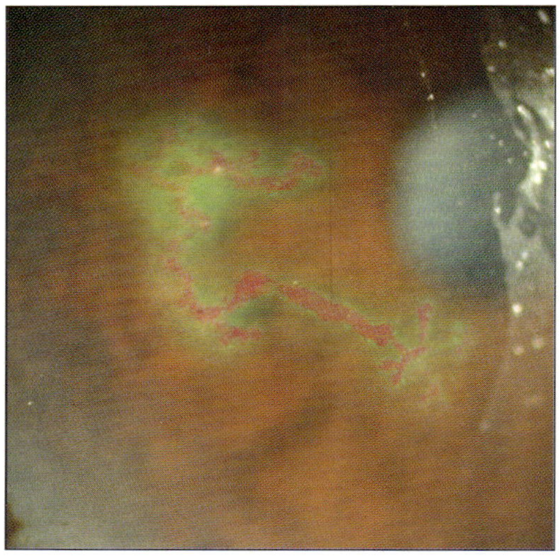

Fig. 2.6: Dendritic ulcer stained with fluorescein with few keratic precipitates

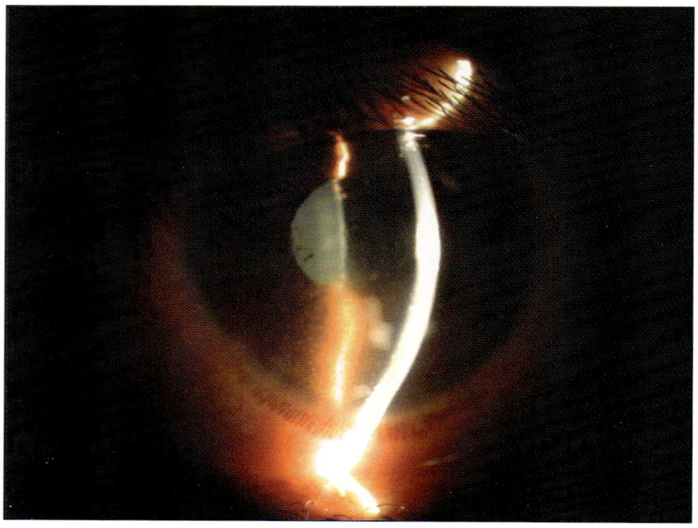

Fig. 2.7: Herpetic keratouveitis with disciform stromal oedema

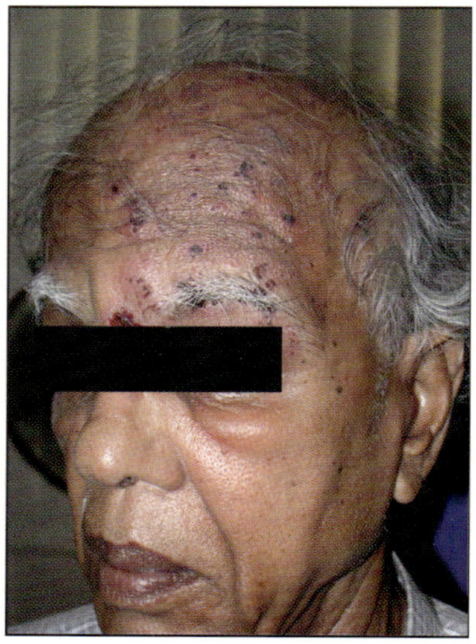

Fig. 2.8: Herpes zoster ophthalmicus with anterior uveitis

CHAPTER THREE

Fuchs' Heterochromic Iridocyclitis

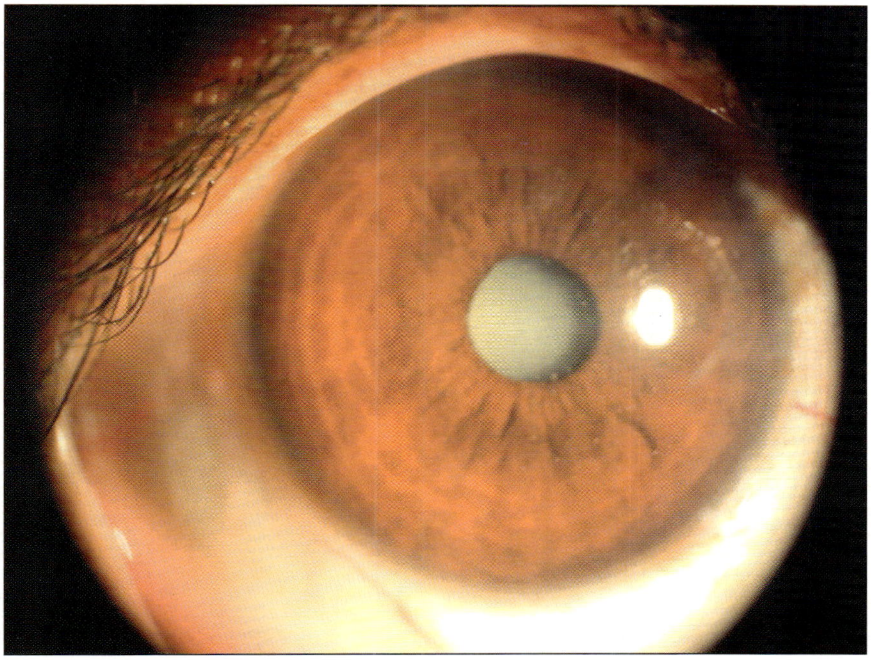

Fuchs' heterochromic iridocyclitis is a chronic, unilateral nongranulomatous anterior uveitis characterized by a white eye, stellate keratic precipitates, iris atrophy with or without iris heterochromia, abnormal angle vessels and absence of posterior synechiae. It is bilateral in approximately 10 percent of patients. The etiology of the disease is still unknown. Several theories including infection from *Toxoplasma gondii,* an immune dysfunction, infiltration of sensitized lymphocytes, and chronic herpetic infection have been proposed.

Ocular Features

Symptoms

Decreased vision due to cataract, floaters due to vitreous opacification.

Signs

- Small, nonpigmented, translucent stellate keratic precipitates with fine filament projections described as stellate scattered over the entire posterior corneal surface.
- Minimal anterior chamber cells and flare.
- Iris heterochromia is present in most patients and usually seen as flattening of the anterior iris features resulting from loss of the anterior iris border layer and iris stroma, especially in the peripupillary area.
- White iris nodules may occur along the border.
- Posterior synechiae are absent. Radial iris vessels are seen on the iris surface because of iris atrophy.
- Fine blood vessels on the trabecular meshwork may bleed when the intraocular pressure suddenly drops during surgery or paracentesis. (Amsler sign).
- Posterior subcapsular cataract
- Vitreous opacification
- Secondary glaucoma is seen in about 60 percent cases

Investigations

Diagnosis is always clinical. No laboratory investigations are required.

Treatment

Topical corticosteroids for the anterior segment inflammation. Cataract and glaucoma are managed with surgery with steroid prophylaxis.

REFERENCES

1. Jones NP: Fuchs' heterochromic uveitis: An update. Surv Ophthalmol 1993; 37: 253-72
2. La Hey E, de Jong PT, Kijlstra A. Fuchs' heterochromic cyclitis: Review of the literature on the pathogenetic mechanisms. Br J Ophthalmol. 1994 ;78:307-12.
3. Velilla S, Dios E, Herreras JM, Calonge M. Fuchs' heterochromic iridocyclitis: a review of 26 cases. Ocul Immunol Inflamm. 2001; 9: 169-75.

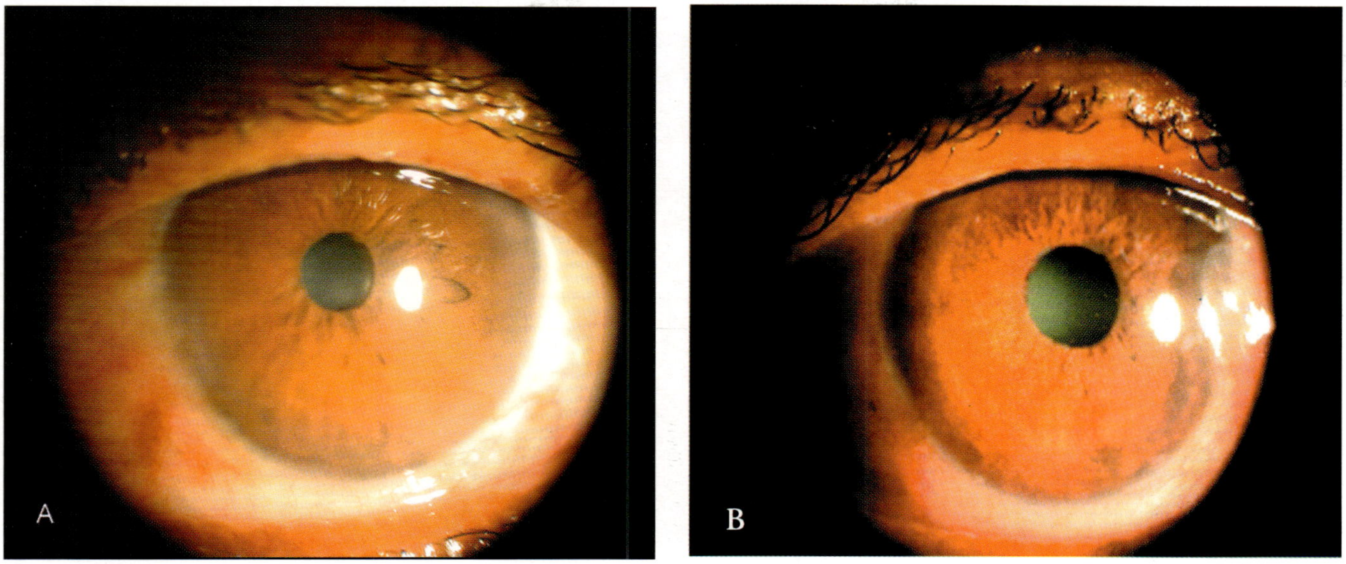

Figs 3.1A and B: Clinical photograph of the right (Fig. A) and left eye (Fig. B) of a 30-year-old man who complained of decreased vision in his left eye for the last 6 months . Slit lamp examination showed diffuse stellate keratic precipitates, pupillary sphincter atrophy, moth-eaten appearance of the iris and posterior subcapsular cataract in left eye. The patient was diagnosed to have Fuchs' heterochromic iridocyclitis

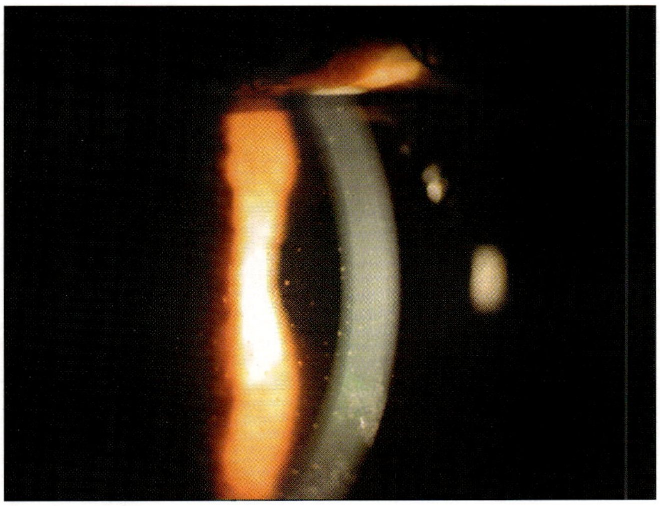

Fig. 3.2: Slit beam photograph under high magnification showing small stellate keratic precipitates with fibrillary extensions

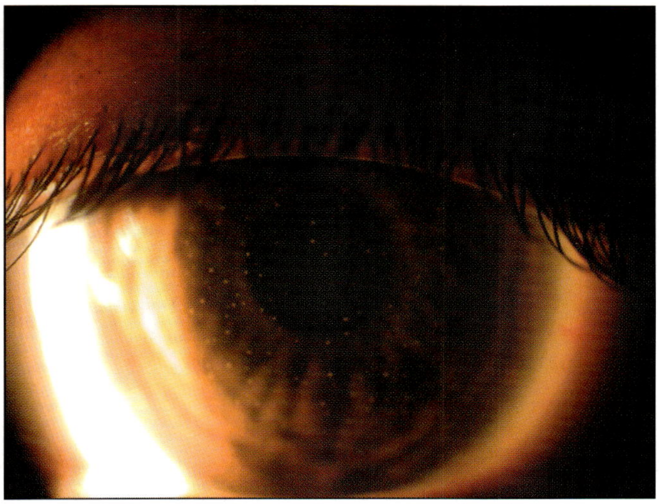

Fig. 3.3: Multiple keratic precipitates spread over entire corneal endothelium in an eye with Fuchs' heterochromic iridocyclitis

CHAPTER FOUR

Juvenile Idiopathic Arthritis (JIA) associated Uveitis

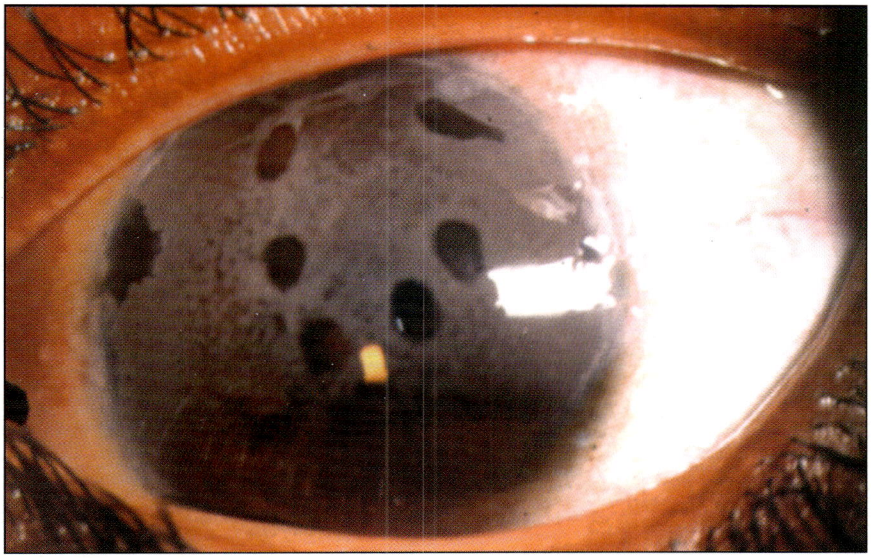

Juvenile idiopathic arthritis (JIA) associated with uveitis is the most frequent cause of chronic intraocular inflammation among children. Chronic iridocyclitis occurs in 10-20 percent of all patients with JIA. Severe loss of vision may occur in 30-40 percent of patients with JIA-associated uveitis. JIA is subdivided into three types.

- Systemic onset JIA (Still's disease)
- Polyarticular onset JIA
- Pauciarticular onset JIA

Ocular Features

Symptoms

Decreased vision.

Signs

- Bilateral nongranulomatous anterior uveitis (70-80%)
- Band keratopathy, small-medium sized keratic precipitates
- Anterior chamber flare
- Posterior synechiae; pupillary membrane
- Posterior subcapsular cataracts
- Vitritis, CME, hypotony maculopathy
- Secondary glaucoma or hypotony late in the disease.

Investigations

- Rheumatoid factor
- Antinuclear antibody (ANA)

Treatment

- Topical steroids: Prednisolone acetate, Betamethasone, Dexamethasone
- Cycloplegic agents: Atropine, Homatropine, Cyclopentolate.
- Periocular/ systemic steroids and immunosuppressive agents are frequently required in JIA-related anterior uveitis in refractory cases or/ and as a steroid-sparing agent.

REFERENCES

1. Kadayofcilar S, Eldem B, Tumer B. Uveitis in childhood. J Pediatr Ophthalmol Strabismus. 2003;40:335-40.
2. Foster CS. Diagnosis and treatment of juvenile idiopathic arthritis-associated uveitis . Curr Opin Ophthalmol. 2003;14:395-98.
3. Kotaniemi K,Sayolainen A, Karma A, Aho K. Recent advances in uveitis of juvenile idiopathic arthritis. Surv Ophthalmol. 2003;48:489-502. Review

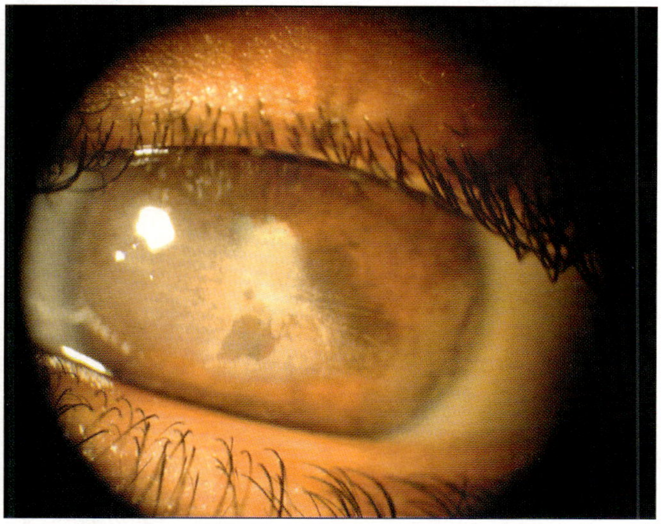

Fig. 4.1: Slit lamp examination of a 10-year-old patient of JIA showing band shaped keratopathy, aqueous cells and flare and complicated cataract

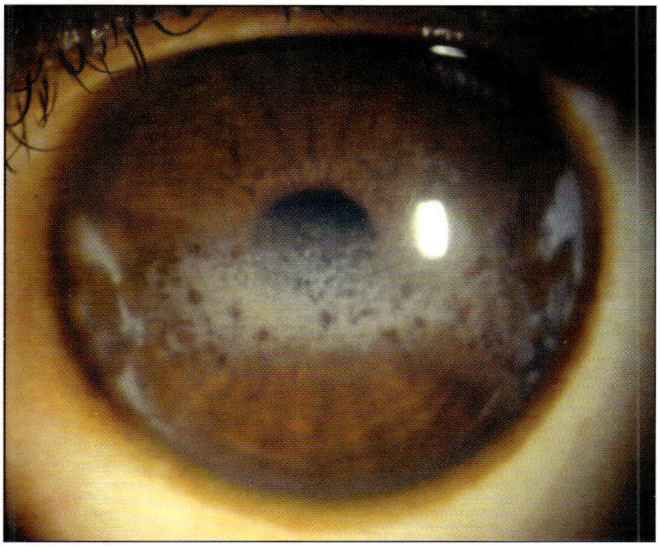

Fig. 4.2: Band keratopathy in juvenile chronic arthritis

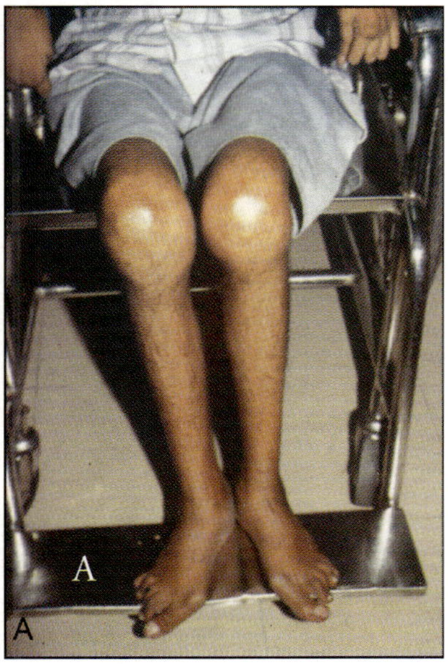

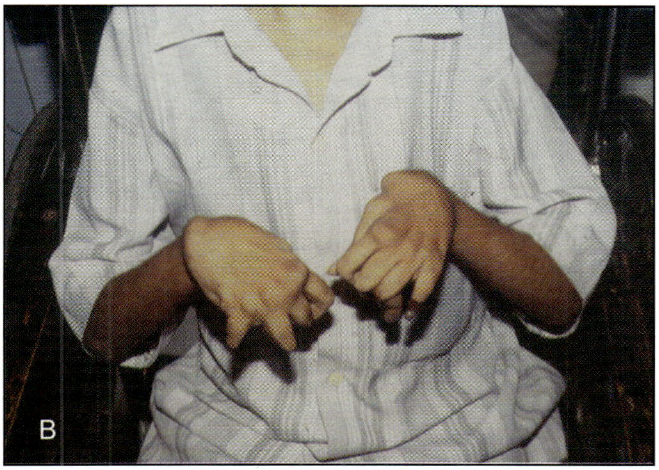

Figs 4.3A and B: Polyarticular onset JIA involving small joints of hand as well as knee, ankle and wrist

CHAPTER FIVE

Lens Induced Uveitis

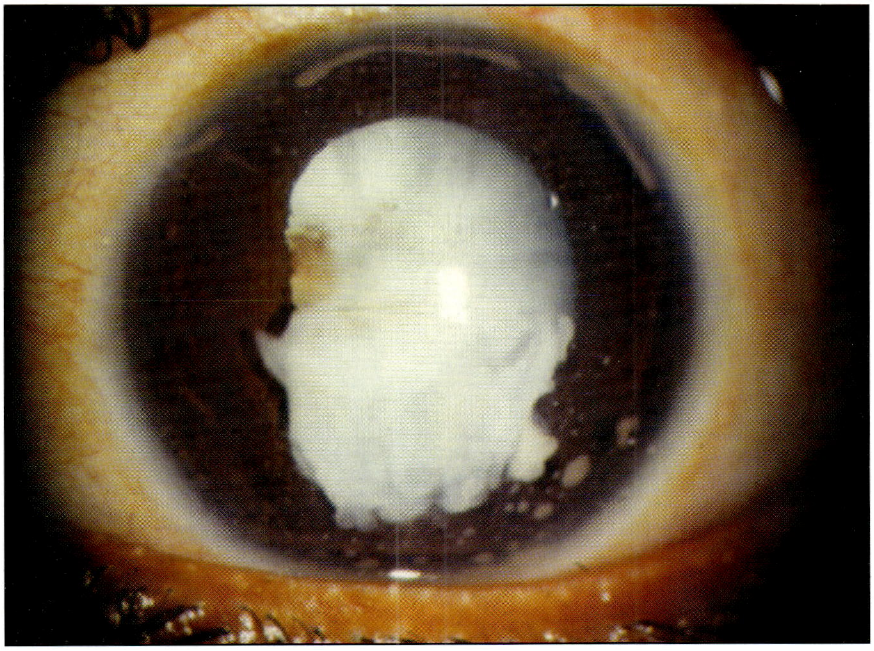

Phacogenic or lens induced uveitis occurs as a result of leakage of lens proteins in hypermature cataract or traumatic cataract or residual cortex after cataract surgery or loss of cortical matter into the vitreous following a posterior capsular rupture during cataract surgery. It is an immunologic response to lens proteins that become autoantigenic upon release into the aqueous humor. Lens induced uveitis may be of two types :

1. Phacoanaphylactic uveitis
2. Phacolytic glaucoma

Ocular Features

Phacoanaphylactic uveitis is a granulomatous inflammation of abrupt onset, presenting with large mutton fat keratic precipitates, thick flare and abundant anterior chamber cells and hypopyon. Lens is opaque with a wrinkled anterior capsule. It occurs days to weeks after surgical or non-surgical disruption of the lens capsule.

Phacolytic glaucoma is an acute glaucoma that occurs in hypermature cataract where lens protein leaks through the capsule and is engulfed by macrophages that obstruct the trabecular meshwork and cause increased intraocular pressure.

Investigations

Aqueous aspirate which shows macrophages engulfed with lens material.

Treatment

Surgical removal of the cataractous lens and the residual lens material.

Topical corticosteroids and cycloplegic agents

REFERENCES

1. Smith RE, Nozik RA:Uveitis : A Clinical Approach to Diagnosis and Management, ed 2.Baltimore:Williams and Wilkins,1989, 198-203.
2. Marak G: Phacoanaphylactic endophthalmitis. Surv Ophthalmol 1992;36:325-339
3. Filipe JC,Palmares J, Delgado L, Lopes JM, Borges J, Castro-Correja J. Phacolytic glaucoma and lens-induced uveitis.Int Ophthalmol 1993;17:289-93.

Lens Induced Uveitis

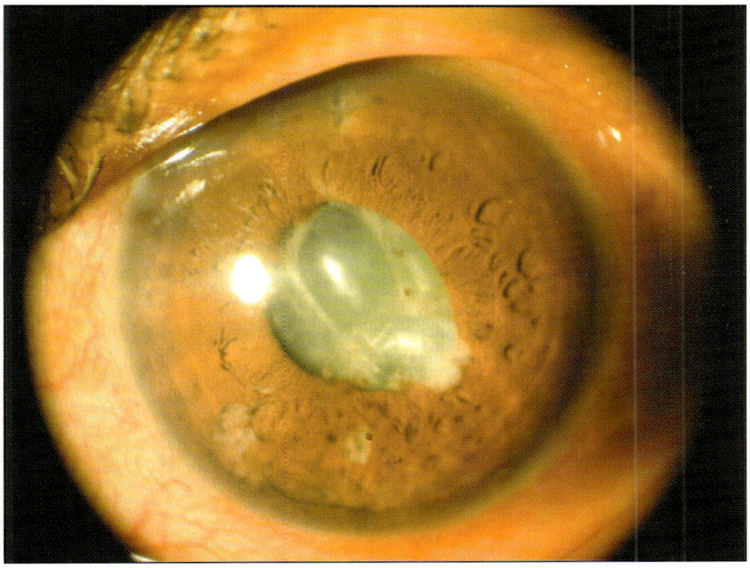

A 45-year-old man complained of pain, redness and decreased vision in his left eye. Past history revealed that he had undergone Nd:Yag sphincterotomy following which he developed cataract

Fig. 5.1: Slit lamp photograph shows aqueous cells and flare , cataractous lens with ruptured anterior lens capsule at 4 o' clock and lens matter in anterior chamber

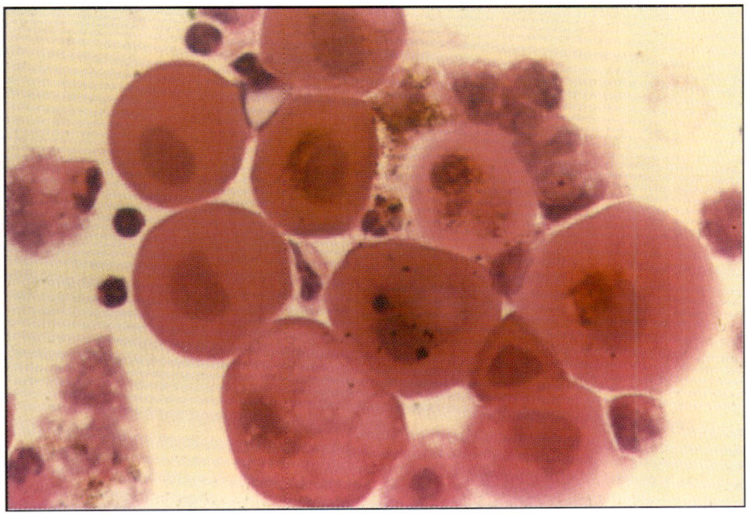

Fig. 5.2: Histopathology showing macrophages engulfing lens material in anterior chamber aspirate of patient with phacoanaphylactic uveitis

CHAPTER SIX

Intraocular Lens Induced Uveitis

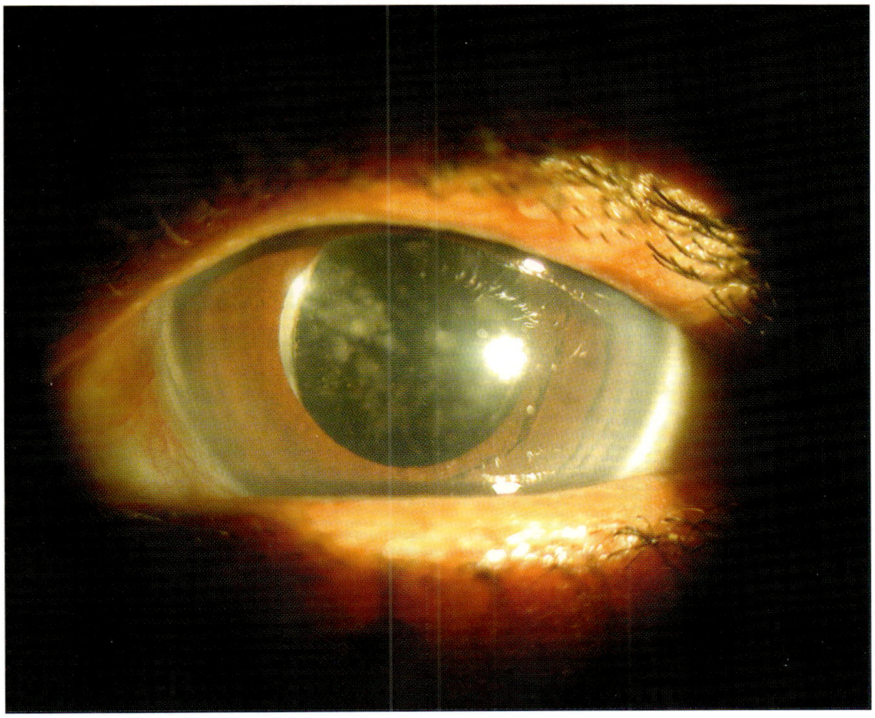

Intraocular inflammation is commonly seen after any intraocular procedure especially after cataract surgery with intraocular lens implantation. Persistent postoperative inflammation can be due to surgical complications or pre-existing uveitis which was uncontrolled. Intraocular lens related uveitis is uncommon these days due to improved lens design and rare use of anterior chamber lenses. Various factors that are responsible for IOL related uveitis are:

1. Position of IOL
   - *Anterior chamber* lenses cause mechanical injury to the iris tissue and angle structures resulting in uveitis, hyphema and elevated intraocular pressure—UGH (uveitis—glaucoma—hyphema) syndrome.
   - *Posterior chamber* (sulcus) Sulcus or scleral fixated lenses erode the ciliary body and cause the breakdown of blood aqueous barrier leading to chronic inflammation.
2. Surface contaminants on the lens surface deposited either during manufacturing process or during surgery may also induce chronic low grade inflammation by releasing inflammatory mediators and activating the complement system.
3. Infection—*Propionobacterium acnes, Staphylococcus epidermidis.*

Ocular Features

Symptoms

Recurrent episodes of pain, photophobia, redness and decreased vision following cataract surgery.

Signs

- Keratic precipitates (small to medium size),
- Mutton fat keratic precipitates in *P. acne* infection
- Aqueous cells and flare
- Hypopyon
- IOL deposits
- Posterior capsule plaque in *P. acne* infection
- Anterior vitreous cells
- Cystoid macular edema.

Investigations

FFA: It shows cystoid macular edema as late hyperfluorescence giving a petalloid appearance to the macula.

UBM: It reveals the location of the haptic of the intraocular lens.

Aqueous aspirate in suspected infections can be investigated for bacteria and fungi using culture and PCR techniques.

Treatment

- Topical steroids, NSAIDs
- IOL polishing using Nd:Yag laser
- Removal of intraocular lens (rare)
- Topical and intravitreal antibiotics in *P. acne* infection.

REFERENCES

1. Carlson AN, Stewart WC, Tso PC. Intraocular lens complications requiring removal or exchange. Surv Ophthalmol 1998 Mar-Apr;42: 417-40.
2. Mamalis N, Nagpal M, Nagpal K, Nagpal PN. Endophthalmitis following cataract surgery. Ophthalmol Clin North Am 2001;14:661-74.
3. El-Harazi SM, Feldman RM. Control of intra-ocular inflammation associated with cataract surgery. Curr Opin Ophthalmol 2001 Feb;12:4-8.

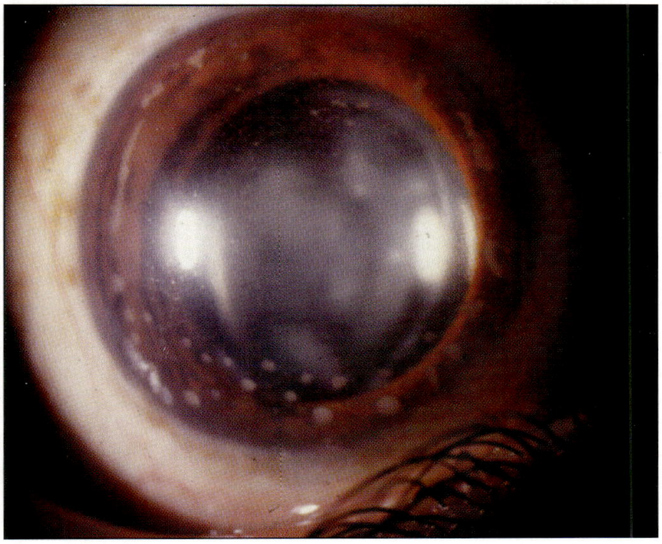

Fig. 6.1: Slit lamp photograph showing granulomatous uveitis with mutton fat keratic precipitates.Exudates are seen behind the intraocular lens. Aqueous tap revealed *Propionibacterium acnes*

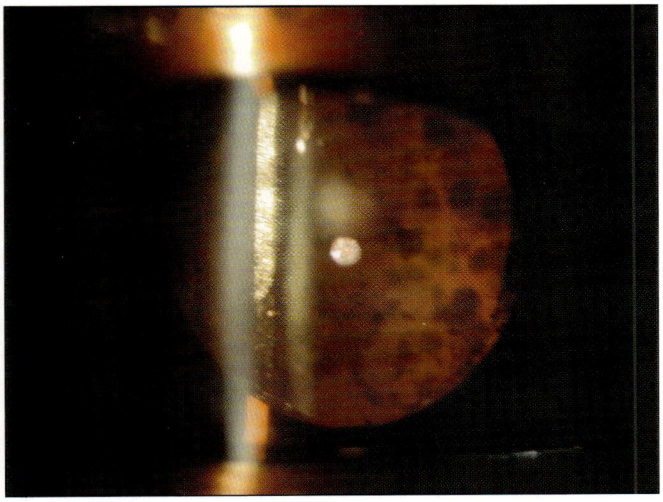

Fig. 6.2: Slit lamp photograph in retroillumination shows large precipitates on anterior surface of the intraocular lens in a case with chronic postoperative inflammation

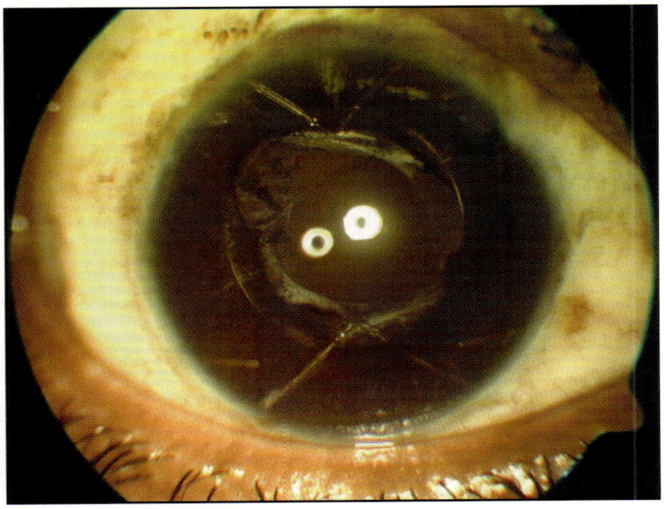

Fig. 6.3: Slit lamp photograph showing anterior chamber intraocular lens which caused recurrent attacks of hyphema due to haptics eroding the iris root and angle structures

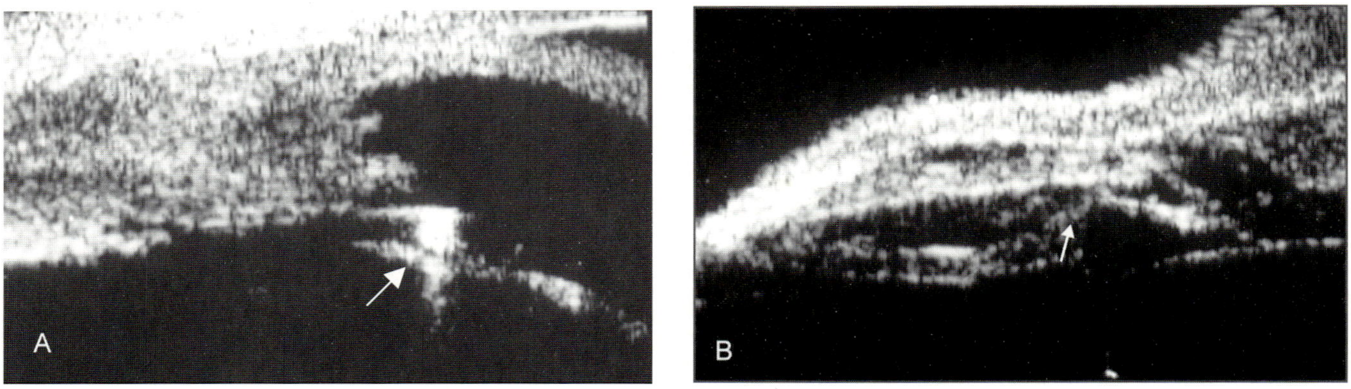

Figs 6.4A and B: Ultrasound biomicroscopy in a pseudophakic eye with chronic inflammation revealed one haptic of IOL inside the bag (arrow) (Fig. A) and the other haptic chafing the iris (Fig. B) thereby causing IOL induced uveitis (arrow)

Section 2
Intermediate Uveitis

CHAPTER SEVEN

Intermediate Uveitis

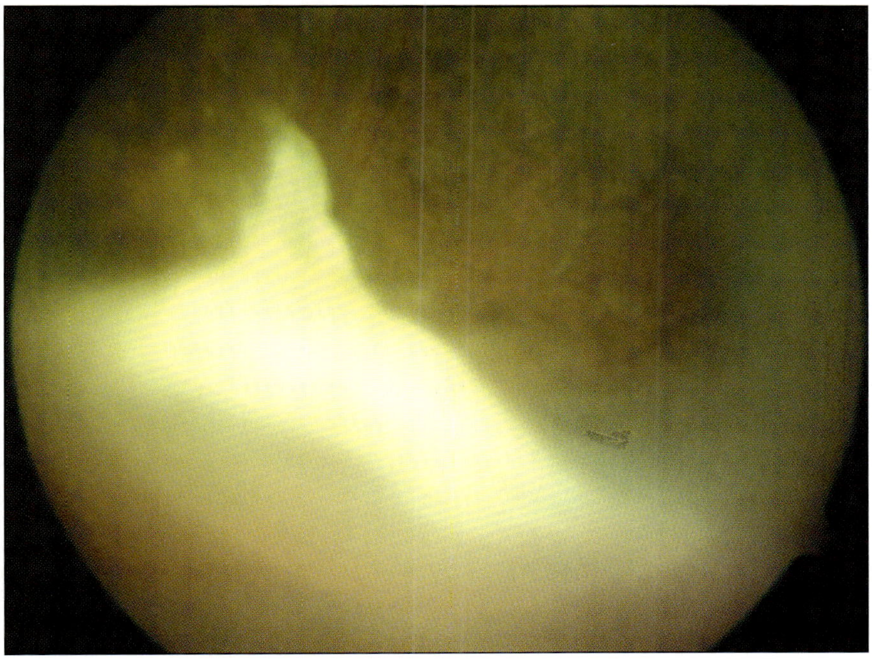

Intermediate uveitis is a term introduced by the International Uveitis Study Group as a part of an anatomical classification for uveitis. Intermediate uveitis is characterized by intraocular inflammation involving the anterior vitreous, peripheral retina, pars plana and ciliary body. It is bilateral in 70-90 percent cases and occurs in patients between the age group of 5 and 40 years. It has a bimodal distribution with a young group between 5-15 years and an older group between 20-40 years. The etiology of the disease is still unknown, however conditions like tuberculosis, sarcoidosis, multiple sclerosis need to be ruled out by relevant investigations.

Ocular Features

Symptoms

Blurring of vision, floaters.

Signs

Anterior segment

- Keratic precipitates, aqueous cells and flare
- Vitreous cells

Posterior segment

- Snowball exudates in the inferior vitreous
- Periphlebitis
- Snow banking in chronic stage
- Neovascularization over pars plana

Complications

- Posterior subcapsular cataract
- Secondary glaucoma
- Cystoid macular edema
- Vitreous hemorrhage
- Retinal detachment and phthisis bulbi.

Investigations

- Complete blood count with differential count
- Erythrocyte sedimentation rate
- Mantoux test
- Serum angiotensin converting enzyme
- Fluorescent treponemal antibody absorption test (FTA-ABS)
- Venereal Disease Research Laboratory Test (VDRL)
- Rapid Plasma Reagin (RPR)
- Chest X-ray

FFA: It shows leakage from the inflamed retinal vessels, optic disc staining and cystoid macular edema.

UBM: It shows pars plana exudates and inflammatory cell aggregates in the pars plana region.

Treatment

Treatment is instituted only for patients with a visual acuity worse than 6/12.

Modified Kaplan Approach

1. Posterior subtenon steroid injection
2. Oral corticosteroids
3. Immunosuppressives
4. Laser photocoagulation or trans-scleral cryotherapy and vitrectomy

REFERENCES

1. Fogla R, Biswas J, Ganesh SK: Evaluation of cataract extraction in intermediate uveitis. Ophthalmic Surgery and Lasers 1999;30:191-198.
2. Biswas J, Raghavendran RS, Vijaya R: Intermediate uveitis of parsplanitis type in identical twins—report of a case. International Ophthalmology. 2000;22:275-278.
3. Lai W W, Pulido J S. Intermediate uveitis: Ophthalmol Clin North Am 2002;15:309-17

Clinical Features of Intermediate Uveitis

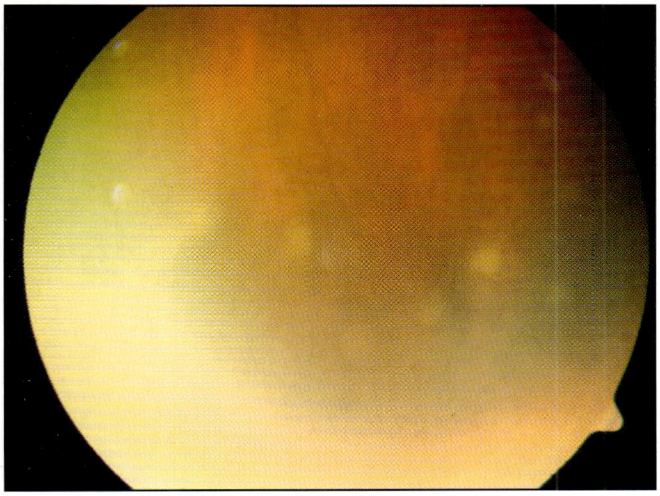

Fig. 7.1: Fundus photograph shows vitreous snowballs in a patient with intermediate uveitis

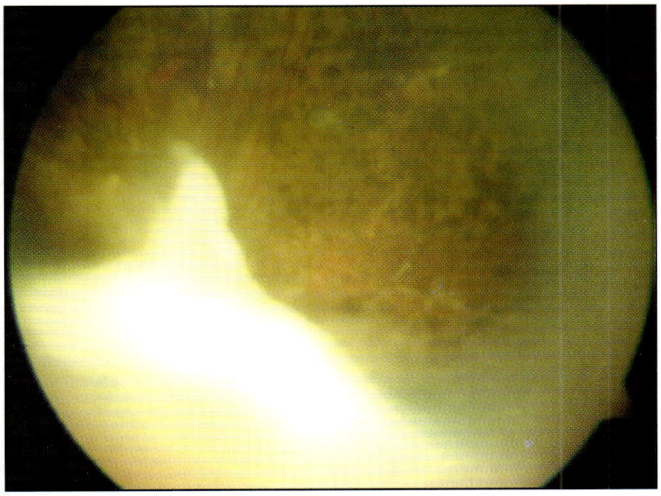

Fig. 7.2: Snow bank formation over the inferior pars plana of a patient with chronic intermediate uveitis

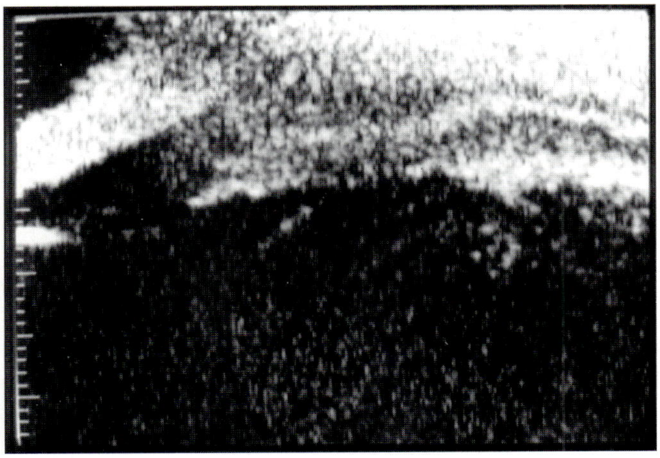

Fig. 7.3: Ultrasound biomicroscopy showing membrane and few dotlike echoes in the pars plana region suggestive of chronic intermediate uveitis

Complications of Intermediate Uveitis

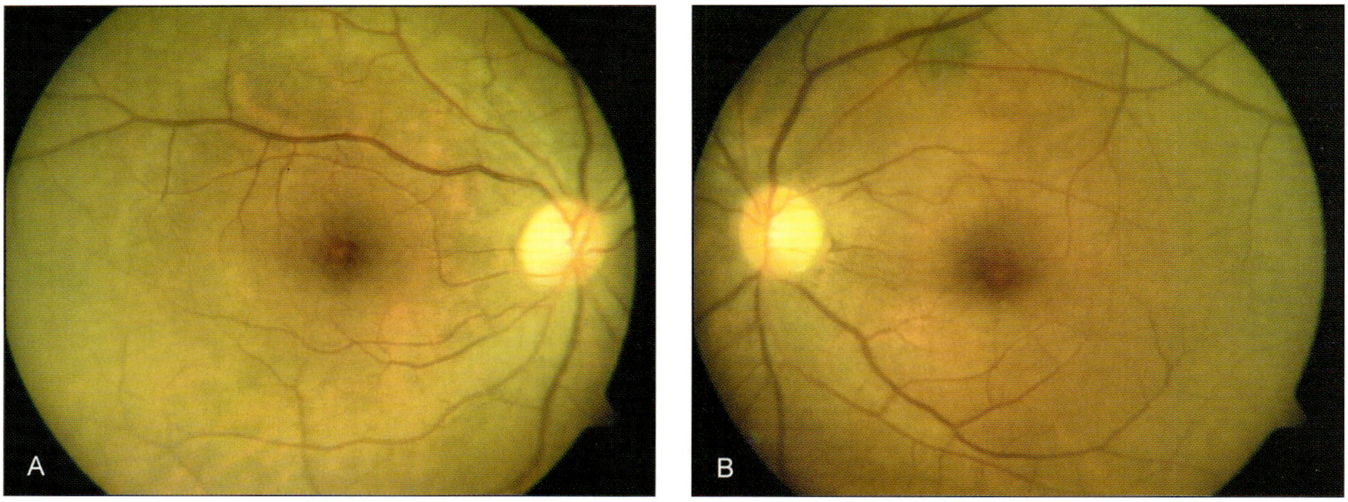

Figs 7.4A and B: A 25-year-old lady presented with complaints of blurred vision since 1 month. Her best corrected visual acuity was 6/9 and 6/12 in the right and left eye respectively. Anterior segment examination was normal. Fundus evaluation revealed vitreous cells and pars plana exudates and cystoid macular edema in both eyes (Figs A and B)

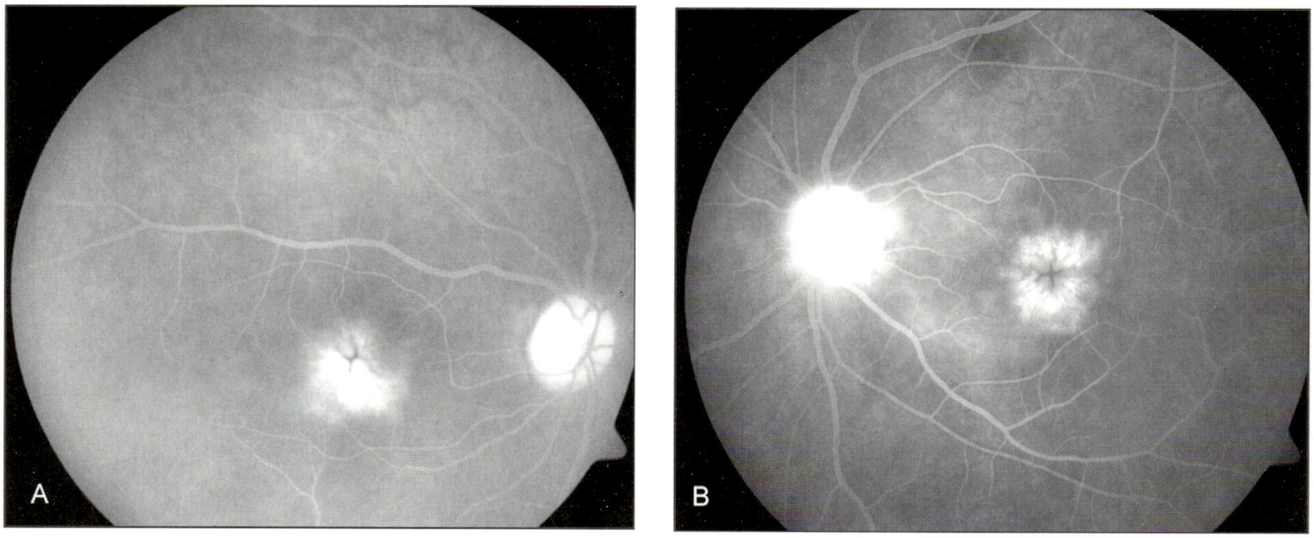

Figs 7.5A and B: Fluorescein angiogram of the same patient in the late phase showed classical petalloid pattern of cystoid macular edema in both eyes

Section 3
Posterior Uveitis

CHAPTER EIGHT

Serpiginous Choroiditis

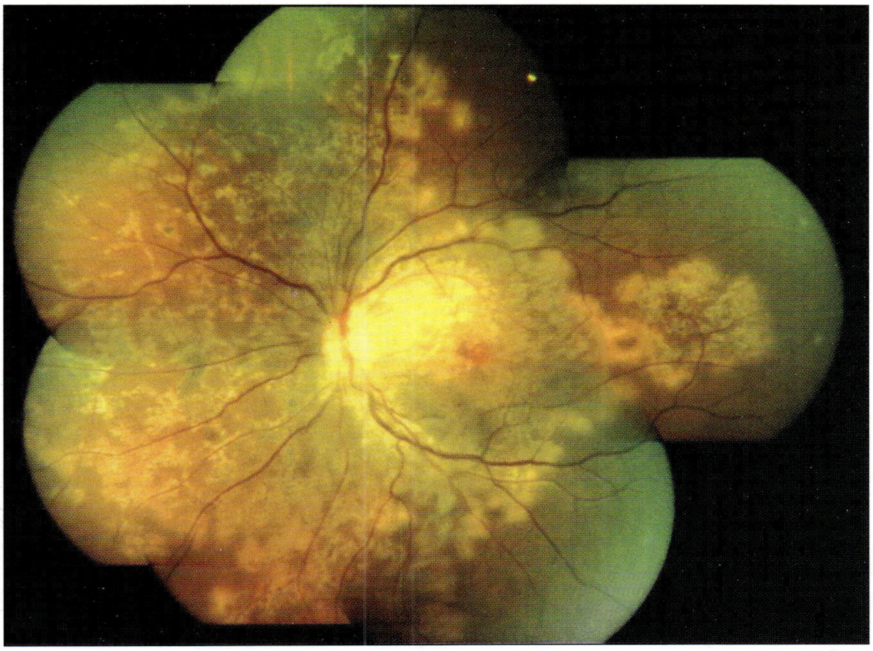

Serpiginous choroiditis is a bilateral, chronic, recurrent, progressive, idiopathic disease affecting the retinal pigment epithelium, the choriocapillaris and the choroid. It is also named as geographic helicoid peripapillary choroidopathy (GHPC).

It affects both sexes equally, commonly during the middle age group. The exact etiology of this disease is not known but recently association with tuberculosis and herpes infection have been reported.

Ocular Features

Symptoms

Blurred vision, metamorphopsia, central and paracentral scotomas

Signs

Gray yellow discoid lesions deep to the retina involving retinal pigment epithelium and choriocapillaris at the juxtapapillary or peripapillary region, progresse centrifugally in an irregular serpentine fashion. Recurrences appear as creamy-yellow subretinal infiltrates at the edges of previous scars. In chronic and recurrent cases of serpiginous choroiditis, choroidal neovascular membrane, serous retinal detachment and areas of chorioretinal atrophy with subretinal fibrosis may be seen.

Macular GHPC

GHPC may present as lesions involving the macula exclusively with a poor prognosis.

Investigations

FFA

- Active stage—Early hypofluorescence with late hyperfluorescence at the border of the lesions.
- Inactive stage—Mottled hyperfluorescence and staining of the scar in the late phase.

ICG

- Early hyperfluorescence with late staining of active lesions.
- Visual field—Absolute scotomas (active lesion), Relative scotomas (resolved lesions).

Treatment

- Oral prednisolone and intravenous pulse methyl prednisolone.
- Immunosuppressives (Azathioprine, Cyclosporine, Mycophenolate mofetil).

REFERENCES

1. Ciulla TA,Gragoudas ES. Serpiginous choroiditis. Int Ophthalmcl Clin 1996;36:135-143
2. Christmas NJ, Oh KT, Oh DM , Folk JC. Long term follow up of patients with serpiginous choroiditis. Retina 2002; 22:550-556.
3. Akpek EK, Jabs DA, Tessler HH, Joondeph BC, Foster CS. Successful treatment of serpiginous choroiditis with alkylating agents. Ophthalmology. 2002;109:1506-13.
4. Quillen DA, Davis JB, Gottlieb JL, Blodi BA, Callanan DG, Chang TS, Equi RA. The white dot syndromes. Am J Ophthalmol 2004; 137:538-550.

Active Geographic Helicoid Peripapillary Choroidopathy

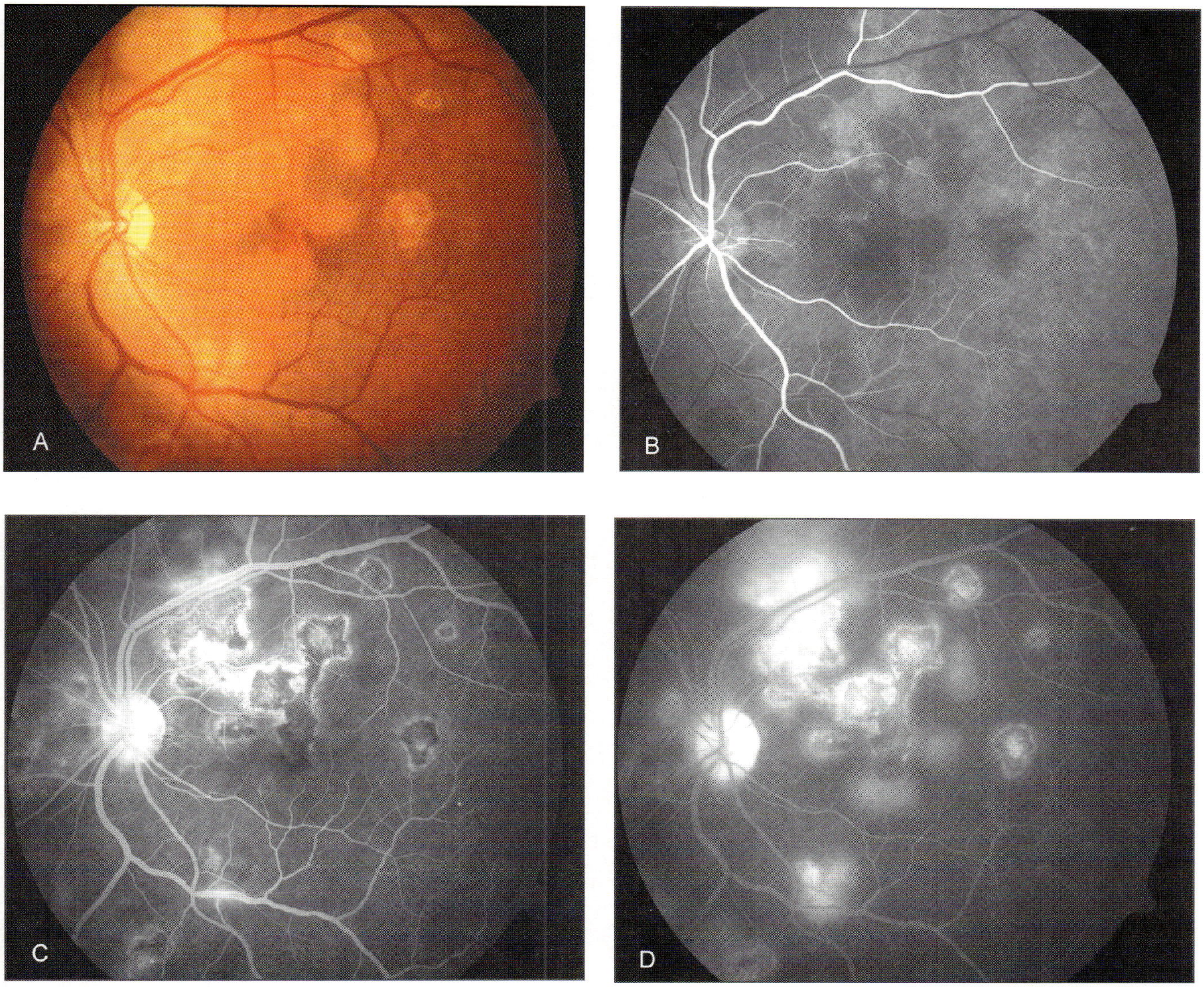

Figs 8.1A to D: (A) Clinical picture demonstrating creamy yellowish lesions in the peripapillary area progressing in a serpentine fashion towards the macular area. (B to D) Early phase (Fig. B) of fluorescein angiogram showing hypofluorescence of the acute lesions which slowly stain in the middle phase (Fig. C). Late phase of the angiogram shows hyperfluorescence with staining of the active edges of the lesions (Fig. D)

Macular GHPC

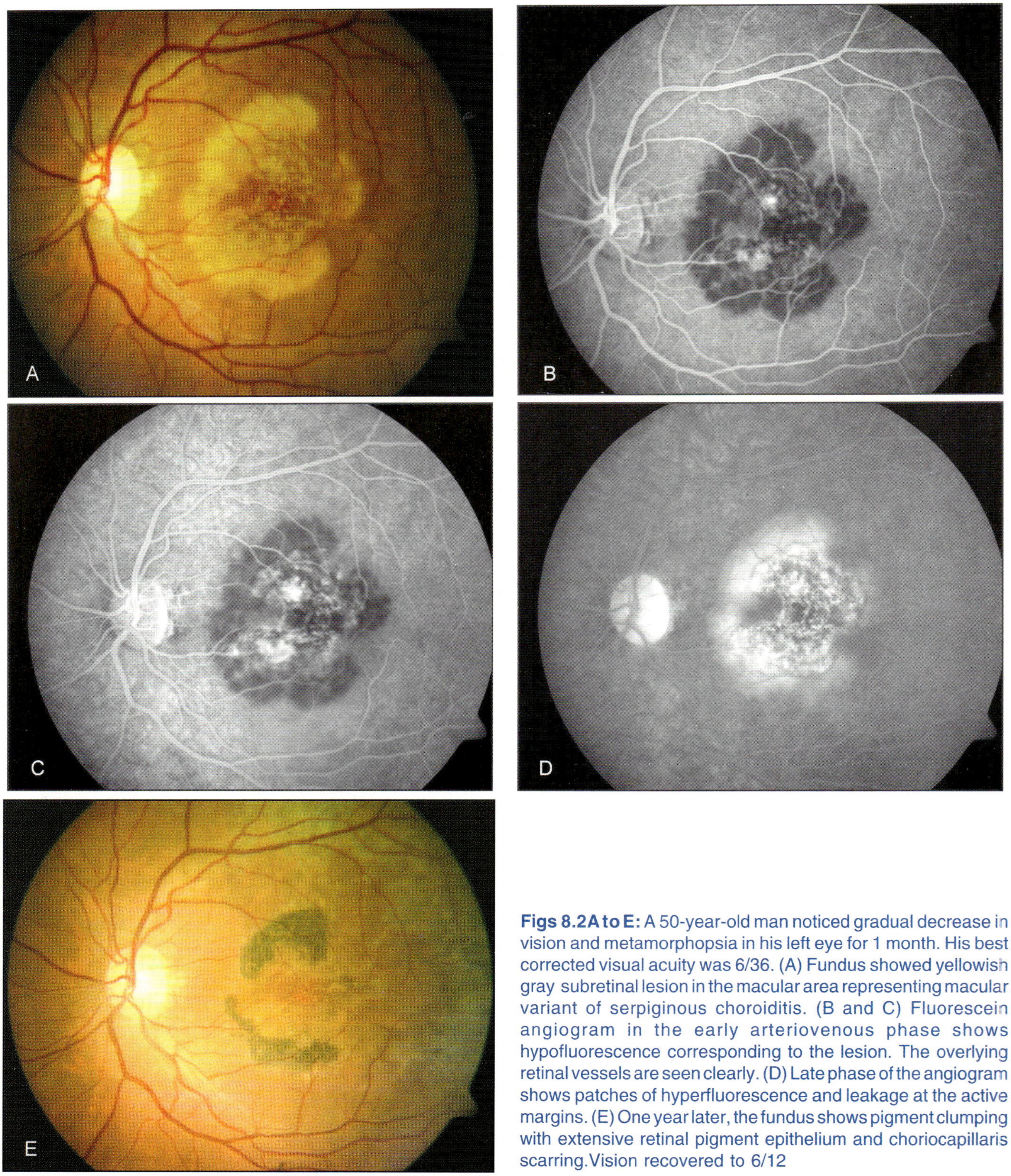

Figs 8.2A to E: A 50-year-old man noticed gradual decrease in vision and metamorphopsia in his left eye for 1 month. His best corrected visual acuity was 6/36. (A) Fundus showed yellowish gray subretinal lesion in the macular area representing macular variant of serpiginous choroiditis. (B and C) Fluorescein angiogram in the early arteriovenous phase shows hypofluorescence corresponding to the lesion. The overlying retinal vessels are seen clearly. (D) Late phase of the angiogram shows patches of hyperfluorescence and leakage at the active margins. (E) One year later, the fundus shows pigment clumping with extensive retinal pigment epithelium and choriocapillaris scarring. Vision recovered to 6/12

Active GHPC

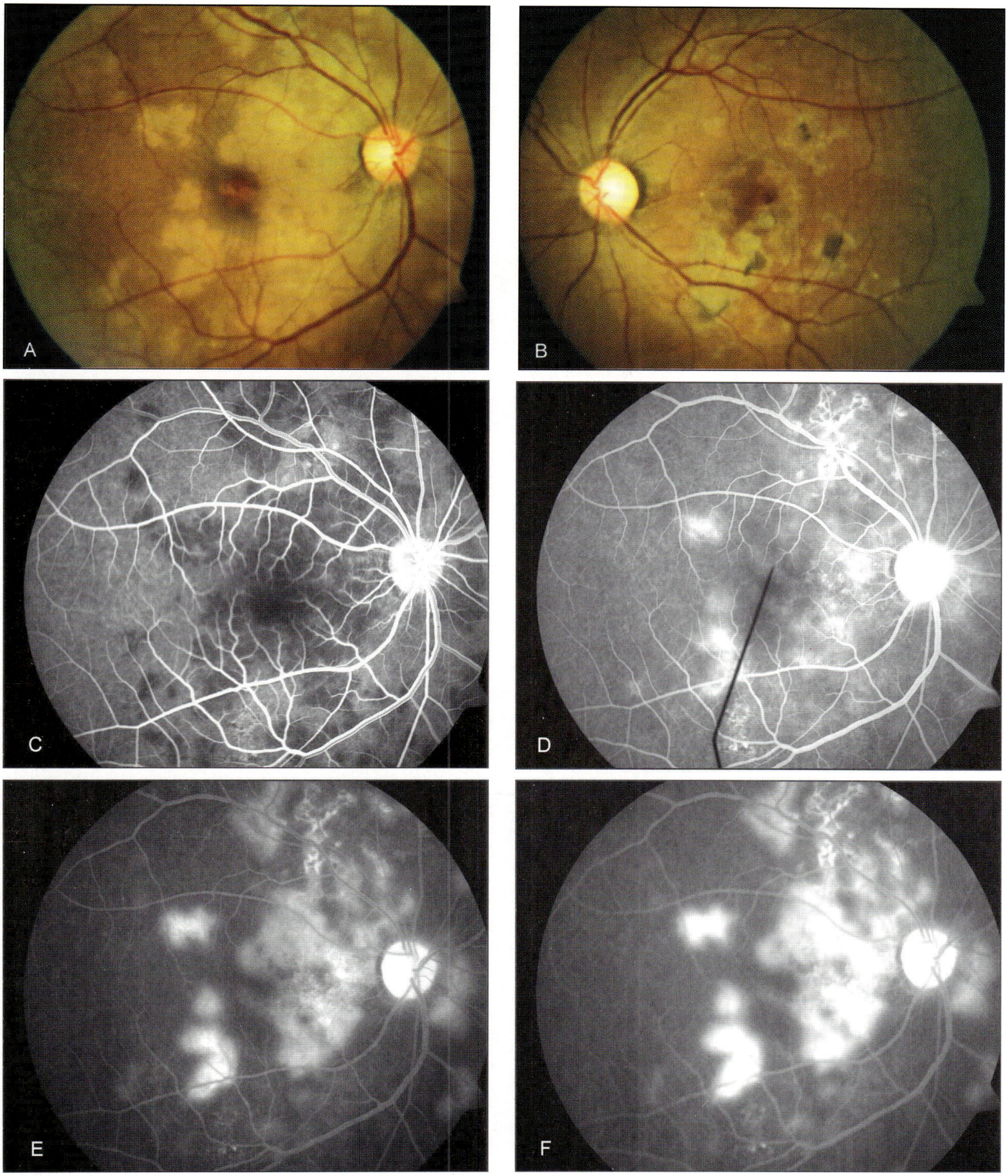

Figs 8.3A to F: (A) Geographic helicoid peripapillary lesions involving the fovea in the right eye of a patient. (B) Left eye of the same patient shows extensive scarring near the disc and macula. (C to F) Fluorescein angiogram of the right eye shows hypofluorescence in early A-V phase followed by hyperfluorescence and staining of the active lesions in late phase

Ampigenous Choroiditis

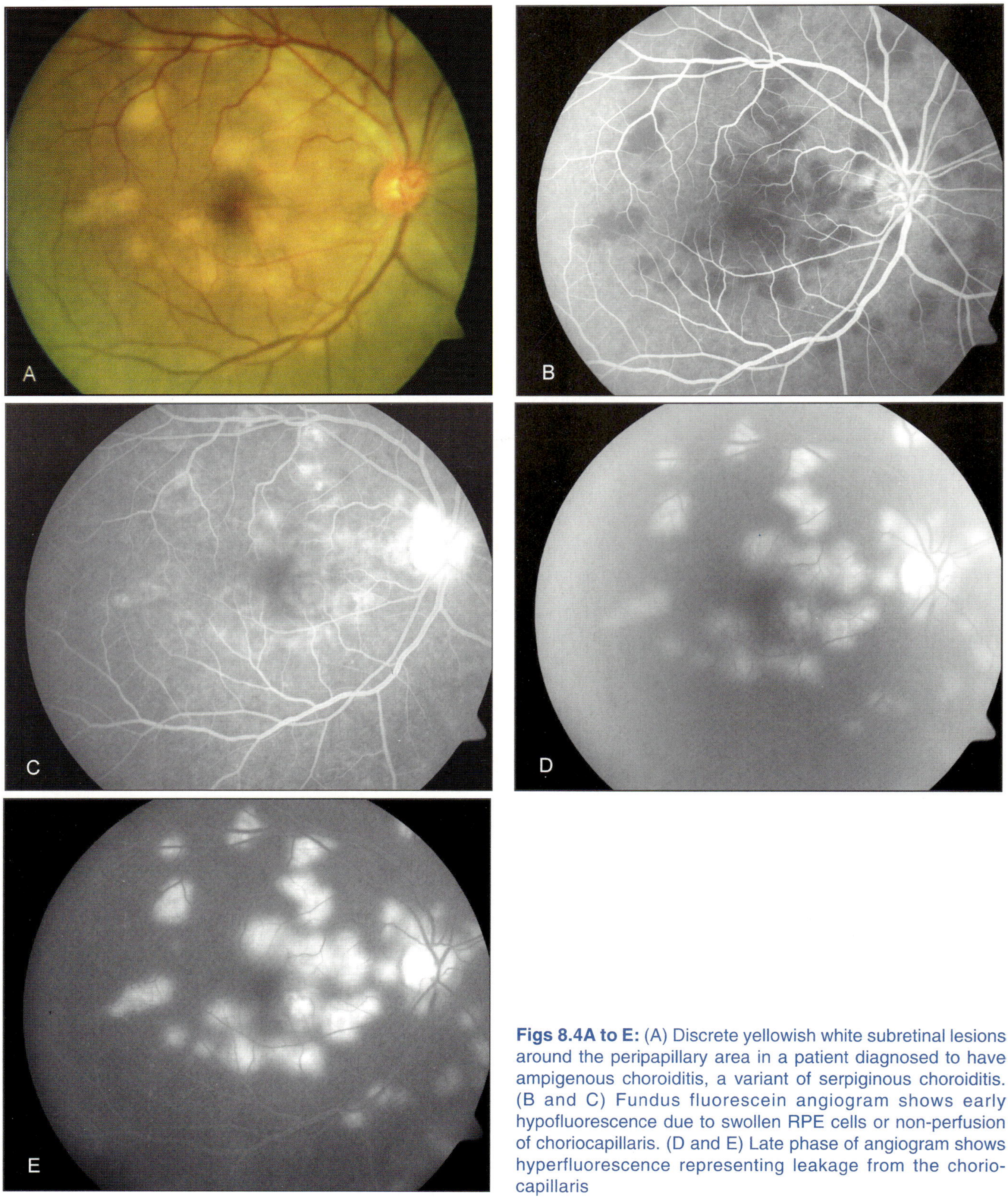

Figs 8.4A to E: (A) Discrete yellowish white subretinal lesions around the peripapillary area in a patient diagnosed to have ampigenous choroiditis, a variant of serpiginous choroiditis. (B and C) Fundus fluorescein angiogram shows early hypofluorescence due to swollen RPE cells or non-perfusion of choriocapillaris. (D and E) Late phase of angiogram shows hyperfluorescence representing leakage from the choriocapillaris

Ampigenous Choroiditis

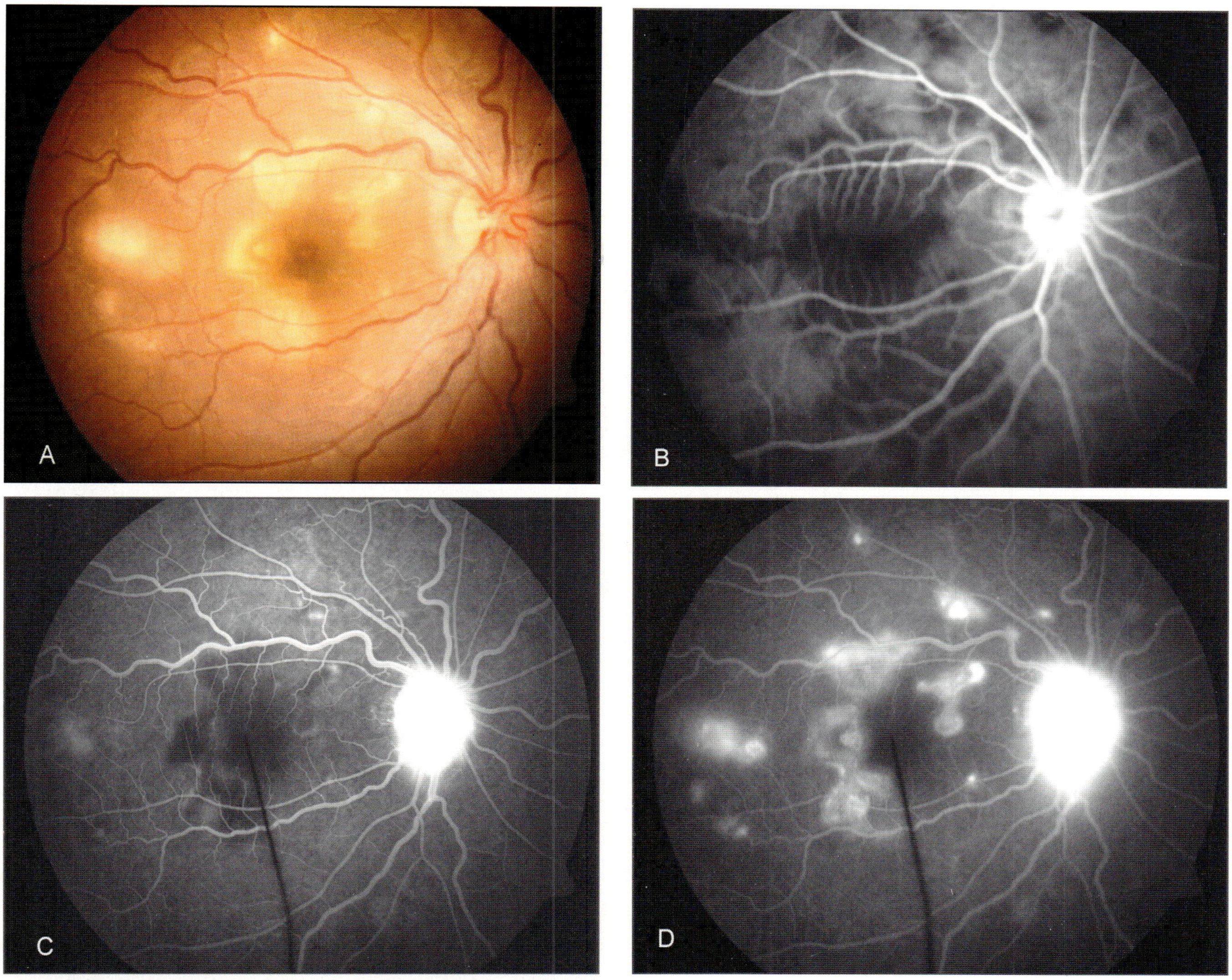

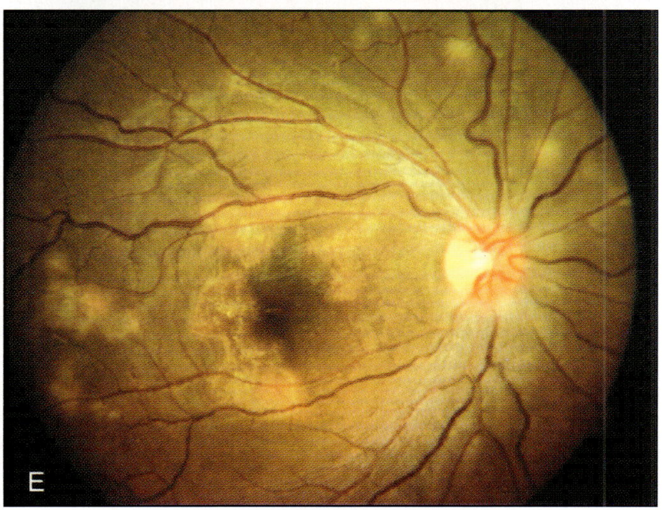

Figs 8.5A to E: (A) Fundus photograph shows multiple yellowish white active choroiditis lesions over the posterior pole and involving the macula. (B to D) Fluorescein angiogram reveals areas of blocked choroidal fluorescence in the early phase and hyperfluorescence and staining in the late phase. (E) Punctate scars with pigment clumping after the resolution of choroiditis

CHAPTER NINE

Multiple Evanescent White Dot Syndrome (MEWDS)

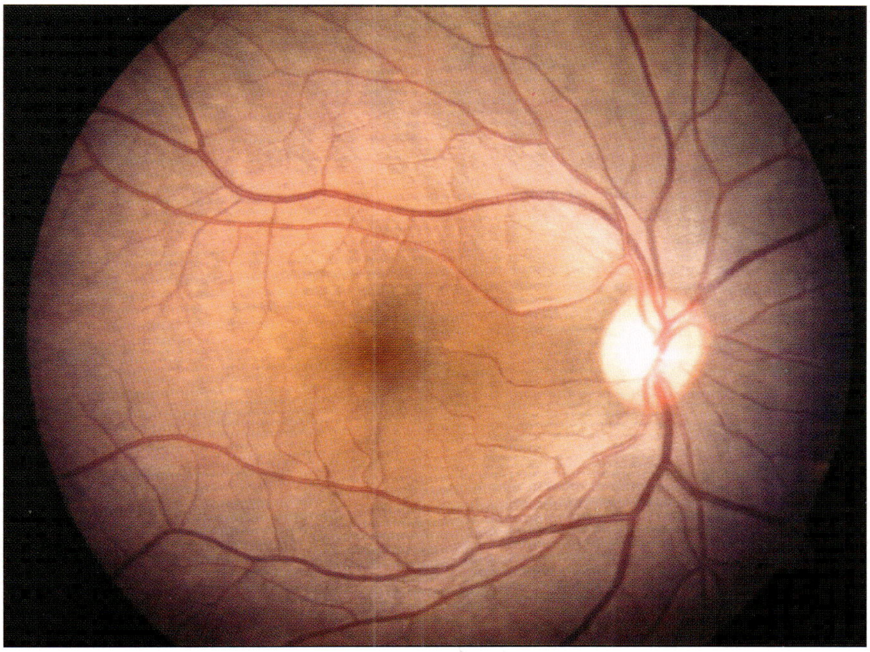

Multiple evanescent white dot syndrome was first reported by Jampol et al in 1984. It is usually unilateral and affects young females in the age group of 17-45 years. The etiology of the disease is unknown but a prodromal viral illness may be associated with the disease.

Ocular Features

Symptoms

Blurred vision, paracentral scotomas, photopsia.

Signs

Anterior segment: Quiet, few vitreous cells

Posterior segment: Numerous small discrete white lesions (100-200 μm) at the level of deep retina and RPE, concentrated perifoveally and over posterior pole extending to the midperiphery. The macula shows a granular appearance with tiny white or light orange specks. Optic nerve head swelling and retinal venous sheathing may also be seen.

The disease is self-limiting and usually heals without scarring. Recurrence is rare.

Investigations

- FFA: Early hyperfluorescence of the white dots with late staining.
- ICG: Multiple hypofluorescent dots all over the fundus.
- Visual field: Enlarged blind spot, central, ceco-central, arcuate scotomas

Treatment

It is a self limiting disease. No treatment is needed.

REFERENCES

1. Jampol LM, Sieving PA, Pugh D et al. Multiple evanescent white dot syndrome. I. Clinical findings. Arch Ophthalmol 1984;102:671.
2. Tsai L Jampol LM, Pollock SC, Olk J. Chronic recurrent multiple evanescent white dot syndrome. Retina 1994;14:160-163.
3. Jampol LM, Wiredu A. MEWDS, MFC, PIC, AMN, AIBSE, and AZOOR: one disease or many? Retina. 1995;15 (5):373-78
4. Quillen DA, Davis JB, et al. Perspective. The White Dot Syndromes. Am J Ophthalmol 2004;137:538-50.

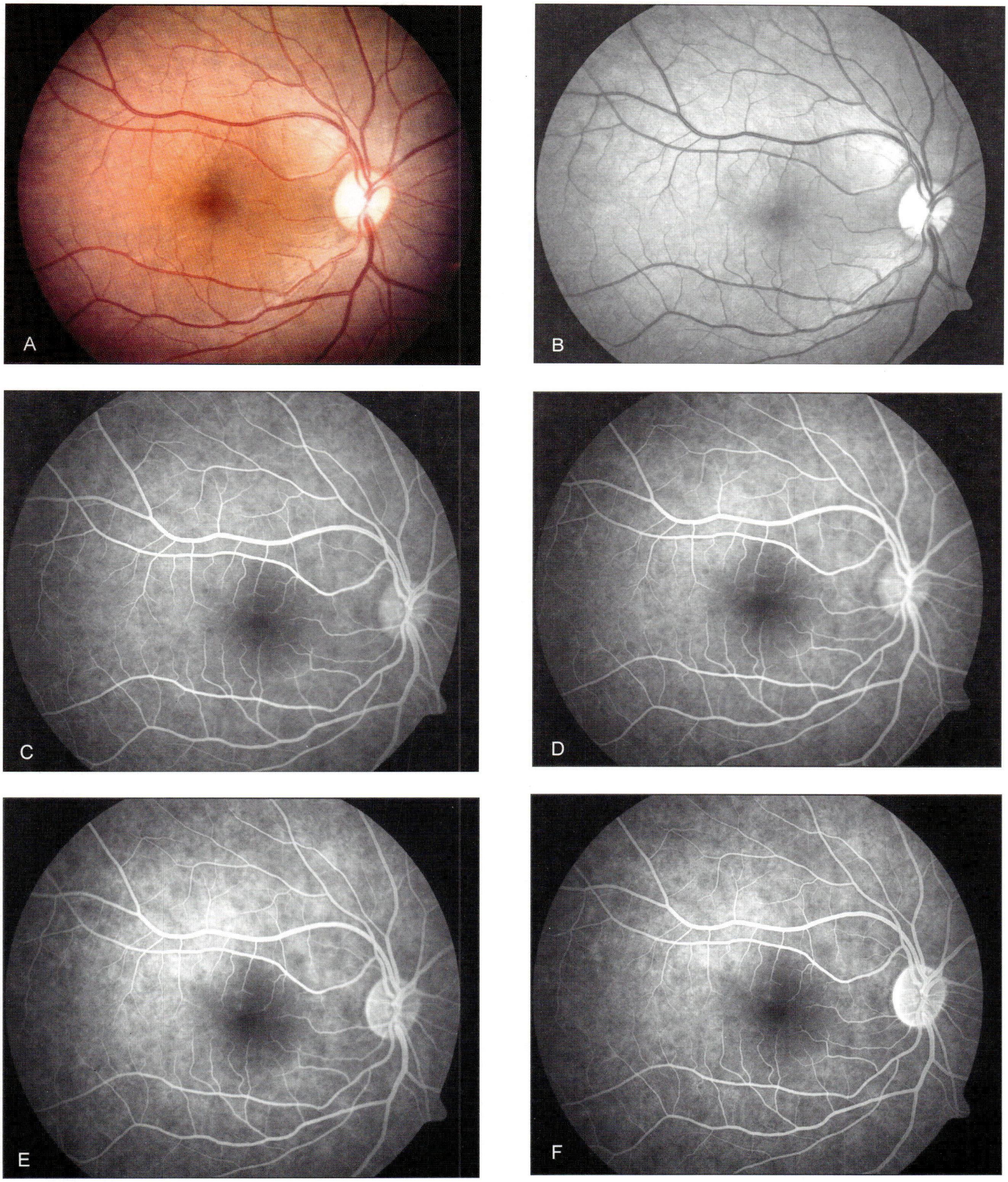

Figs. 9.1A to F: (A) Fundus photograph of a patient with MEWDS showing subtle, yellowish white, granular, deep retinal or RPE lesions in the posterior pole. (B) Red free photograph corresponding to the clinical photograph. (C to F) Fluorescent angiogram shows early hyperfluorescence of white dots with staining in the late phase of the angiogram

CHAPTER TEN

Acute Posterior Multifocal Placoid Pigment Epitheliopathy (APMPPE)

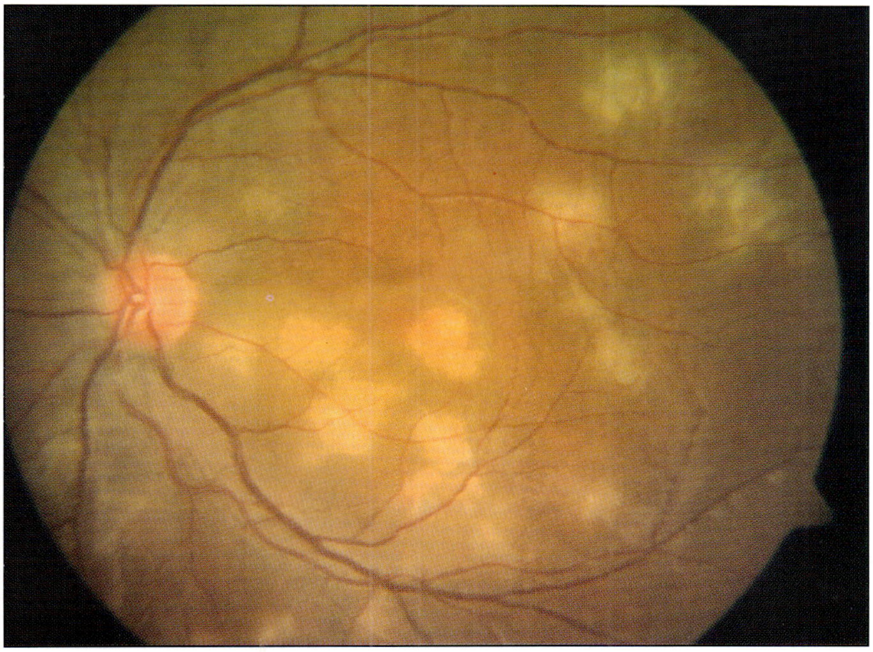

Gass initially described APMPPE in 1968. It is bilateral and affects young adults between 20 and 30 years. Both sexes are equally affected. The etiology of the disease is unknown. It has been postulated that an immune mediated reaction to antigens from different pathogens (viruses), result in choroidal vasculitis with secondary changes in the retinal pigment epithelium. Various systemic conditions associated with APMPPE are cerebral vasculitis, sarcoidosis, nephritis and Crohn's disease.

Ocular Features

Symptoms

Painless diminution of vision

Signs

- Anterior segment: Usually quiet with few vitreous cells
- Posterior segment: Multiple placoid cream colored lesions at the level of RPE in the posterior pole. These lesions heal with RPE mottling, depigmentation or scarring. The disease is often self-limiting.

Complications

Choroidal neovascular membrane/serous RD.

Investigations

- FFA: Early hypofluorescence followed by late hyperfluorescence due to leakage of the dye from the choroid into the damaged retinal pigment epithelial cells.
- ICG: Marked choroidal hypofluorescence in both early and late phase.

Treatment

It is a self-limiting disease. Steroids and rarely immunosuppressives are used when required.

REFERENCES

1. Gass JDM. Acute posterior multifocal placoid pigment epitheliopathy. Arch Ophthalmol 1968;80:177-85.
2. Jones NP: Acute posterior multifocal placoid pigment epitheliopathy. Br J Ophthalmol 1995; 79 (4): 384-89.
3. Quillen DA, Davis JB, et al. Perspective. The White Dot Syndromes. Am J Ophthalmol 2004;137:538-50.

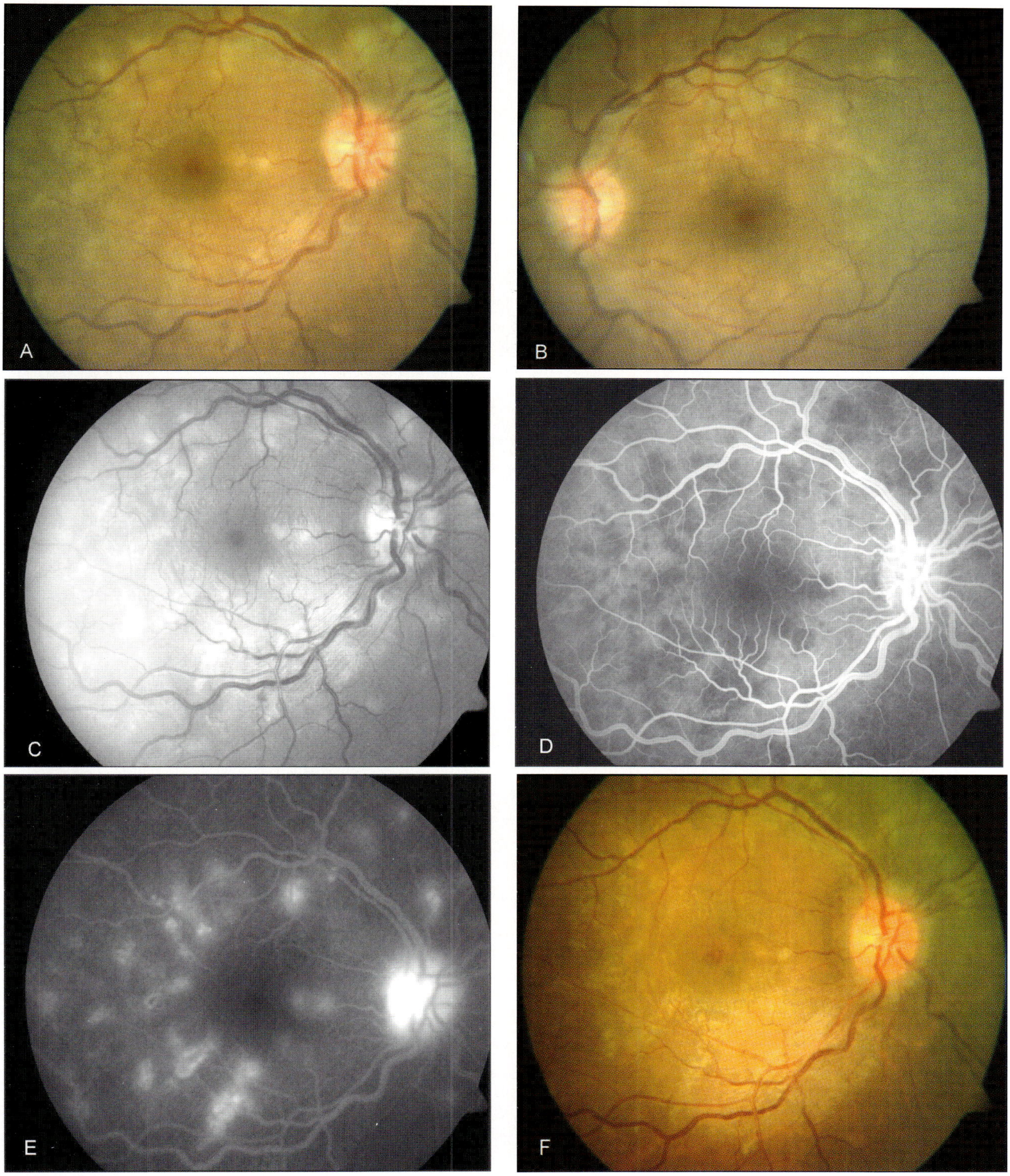

Figs 10.1A to F: (A and B) Fundus photos show multiple round, flat, yellowish white subretinal lesions involving the posterior pole in the right and left eye of an 18-year-old patient who presented with acute diminution of vision. (C and D) Fluorescein angiogram of right eye demonstrates early hypofluorescence due to RPE swelling and choroidal ischemia. (E) Late phase shows hyperfluorescence resulting from leakage of the dye from the choroid into the RPE cells. (F) RPE alterations after the resolution of inflammation when vision recovered to 6/6

CHAPTER ELEVEN

Birdshot Retinochoroidopathy

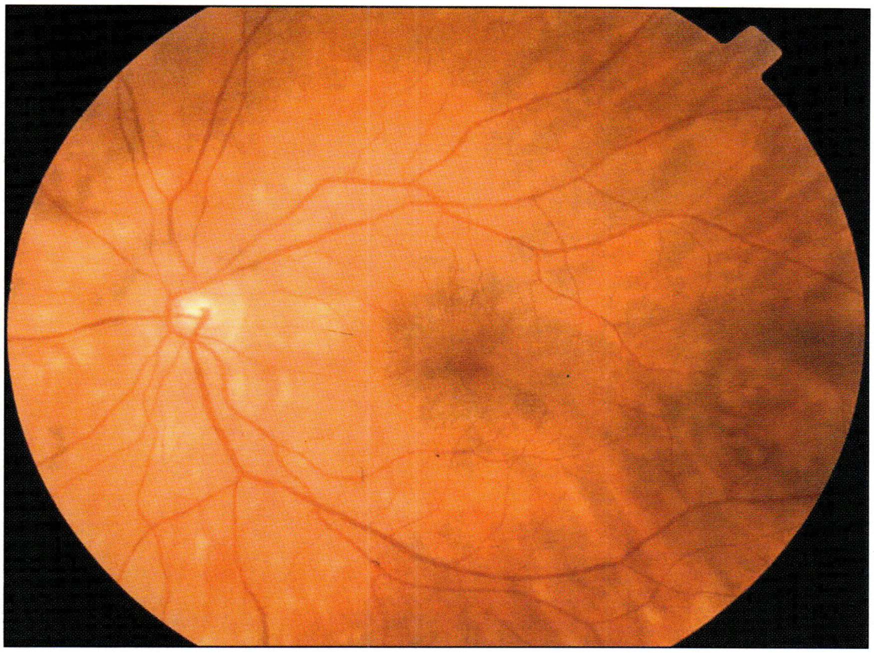

Ryan and Maumenee first described Birdshot choroidopathy in 1980. It is an idiopathic entity associated with HLA-A 29 positivity. It is an asymmetric bilateral disease seen in elderly females between 30-70 years of age.

Ocular Features

Symptoms

Gradual painless loss of vision, floaters

Signs

- *Anterior segment:* Nongranulomatous anterior uveitis. Diffuse vitritis without pars plana exudates.
- *Posterior segment:* Multiple ovoid cream colored lesions 50-1500 μm in size located postequatorially and oriented radially along the large choroidal vessels. These lesions are at the level of outer retina, RPE and inner choroid.

  Disc edema, venous sheathing and CME are often present.

Complications

1. Choroidal neovascular membrane
2. Optic atrophy
3. Serous retinal detachment
4. CME

Investigations

- HLA: A 29 typing
- FFA: Early hypofluorescence of the cream colored lesions with staining in the late phase. Hyperfluorescence of the optic disc and cystoid macular edema in the form of petalloid hyperfluorescence.
- ICG: Multiple hypofluorescent spots much more in number than seen clinically on fluorescein angiography.

Treatment

- Periocular and systemic steroids
- Immunosuppressives (Cyclosporine) in recalcitrant cases.

REFERENCES

1. Ryan SJ, Maumenee AE. Birdshot retinochoroidopathy. Am J Ophthalmol. 1980;89:31-45.
2. Gasch AT, Smith JA, Whitcup SM. Birdshot retinochoroidopathy. Br J Ophthalmol. 1999;83:241-249.
3. Levinson RD, Gonzales CR. Birdshot retinochoroidopathy: immunopathogenesis, evaluation, and treatment. Ophthalmol Clin North Am. 2002;15:343-350.
4. Quillen DA, Davis JB, et al. Perspective. The White Dot Syndromes. Am J Ophthalmol 2004;137:538-550.

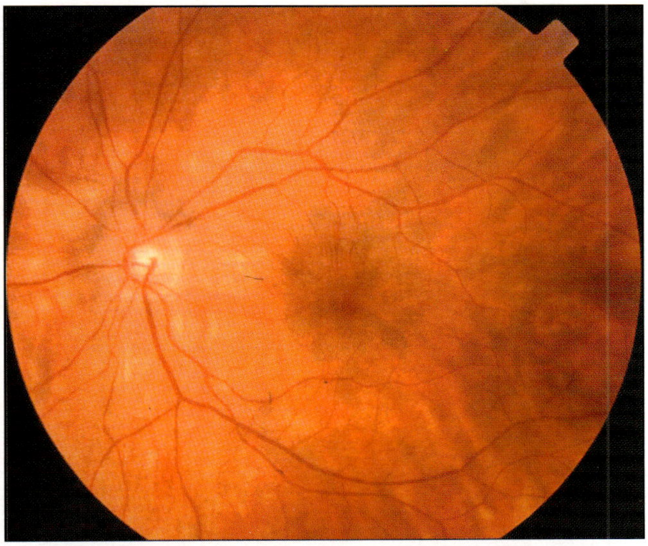

Fig. 11.1: Fundus photograph showing scattered cream colored lesions in the posterior pole in a case of birdshot retinochoroidopathy (*Courtesy* Dr Narsing Rao)

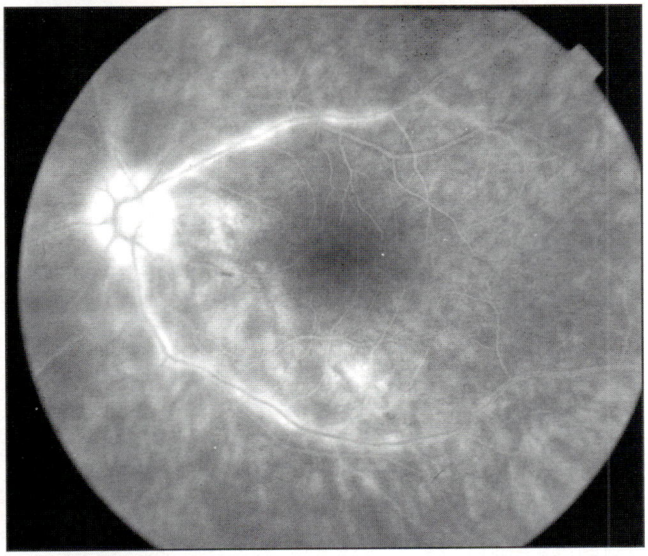

Fig. 11.2: Fluorescein angiogram showed hyperfluorescence of the optic disc and dye leakage from the retinal vessels in the late phase resulting in cystoid macular edema (*Courtesy* Dr Narsing Rao)

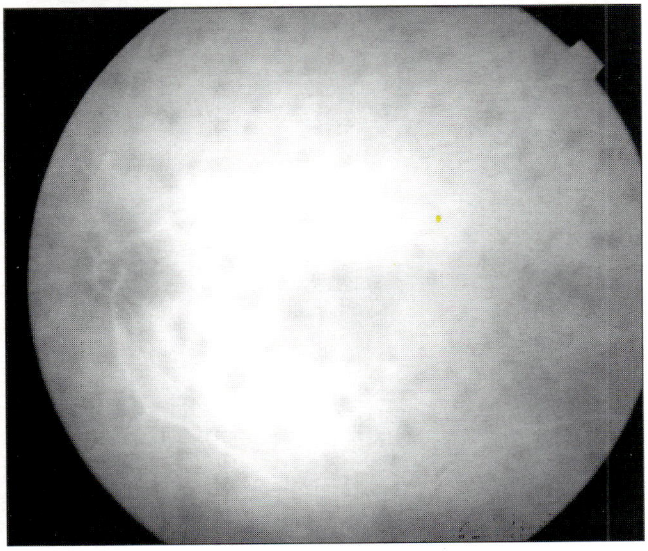

Fig. 11.3: Indocyanine Green Angiography showed numerous hypofluorescent choroidal spots suggestive of hypoperfusion of choriocapillaris (*Courtesy* Dr Narsing Rao)

CHAPTER TWELVE

Punctate Inner Choroidopathy (PIC)

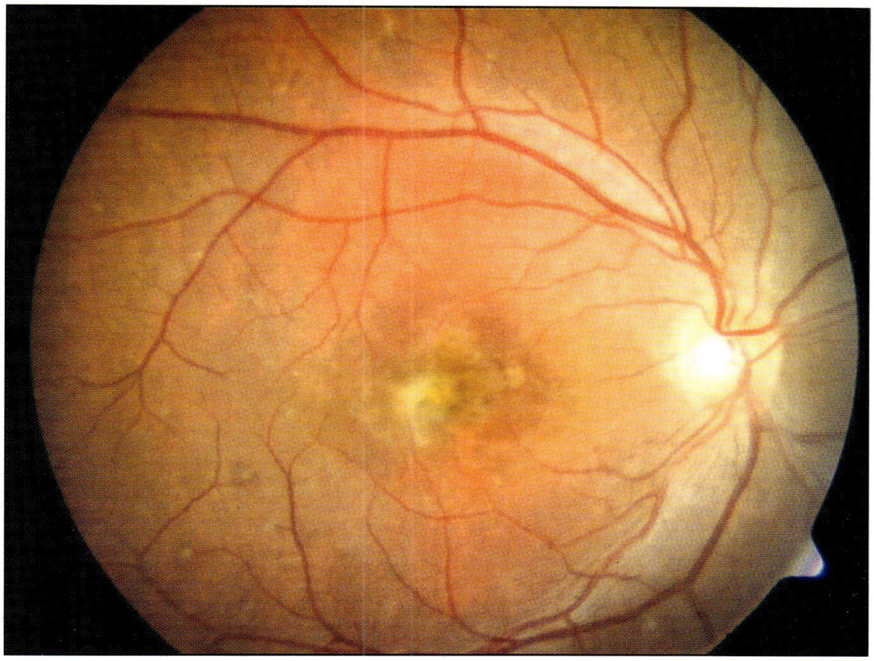

Watzke *et al* first reported PIC in 1984. It is a bilateral entity, commonly seen in young and middle aged myopic women.

Ocular Features

Symptoms

Blurred central vision, central or paracentral scotomas, flashes of light.

Signs

Anterior segment: Quiet and no vitreous inflammation
Posterior segment: Multiple small discrete yellow spots (50-300 μm) at the level of RPE and inner choroid. There may be minimal subretinal fluid overlying the lesion. There is no disc or macular edema. Within weeks, the lesions begin to atrophy and eventually become punched out followed by pigmentation.

Complications

Choroidal neovascular membrane.

Investigations

FFA: Early hyperfluorescence with leakage in the late phase.

ICG: Multiple hypofluorescent dots in the posterior pole.

Visual field: Enlarged blind spot and central scotomas.

Treatment

- No treatment is needed in PIC unless a subretinal neovascular membrane threatens the fovea.

REFERENCE

1. Watzke RC, Packer AJ, Folk JC, et al. Punctate inner choroidopathy. Am J Ophthalmol 1984;98:572-84.

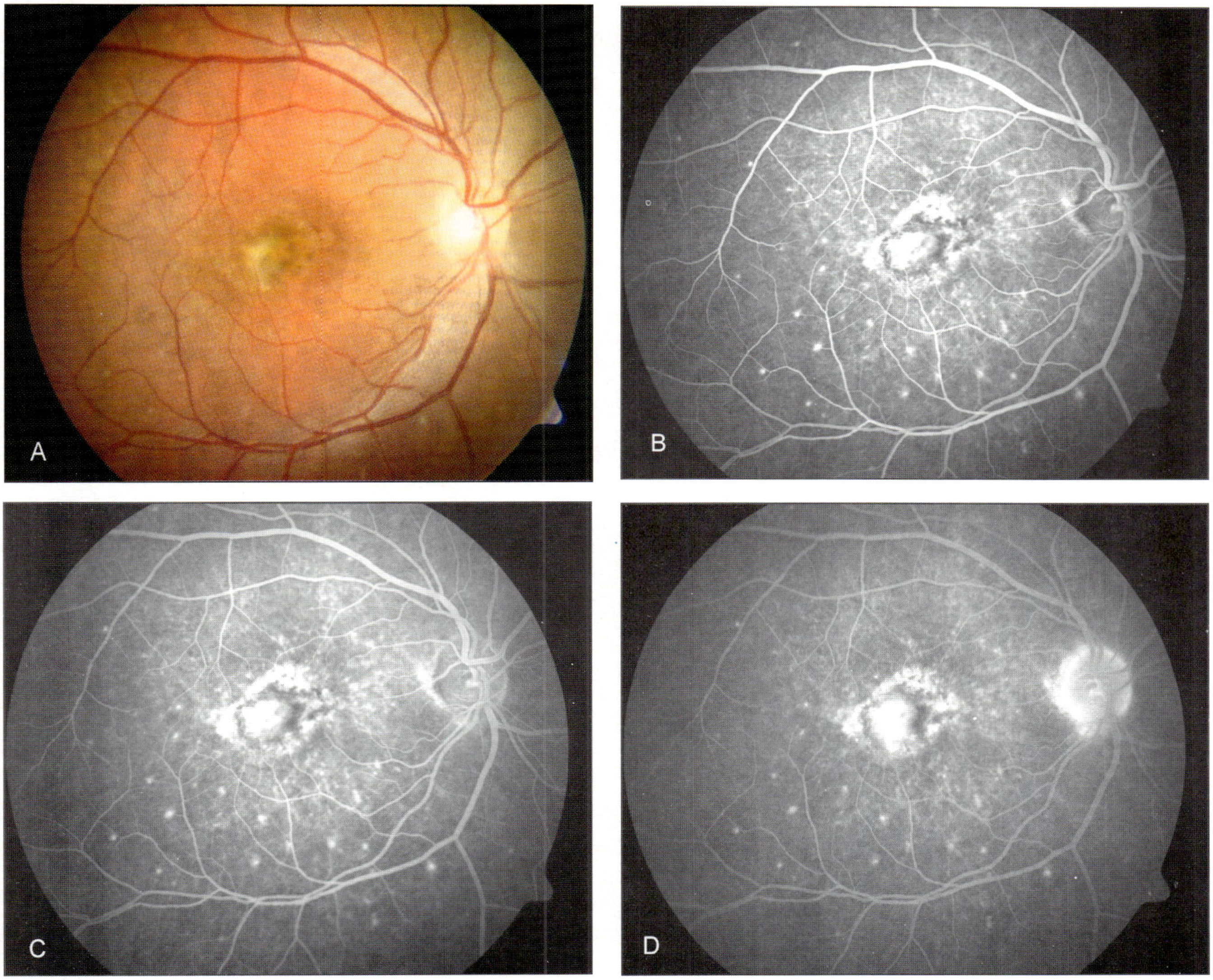

Figs 12.1A to D: A 32-year-old woman complained of blurred vision and metamorphopsia in right eye for 2 weeks. (A) Fundus examination showed punctate white chorioretinal lesions in the posterior pole. A fibrovascular CNVM was also seen at the fovea. (B to D) Fluorescein angiogram in the early phase showed multiple punctate hyperfluorescent lesions with early staining of choroidal neovascular membrane. Late phase of the angiogram revealed staining of the CNVM and fading of the hyperfluorescence of the punctate lesions

CHAPTER THIRTEEN

Choroiditis

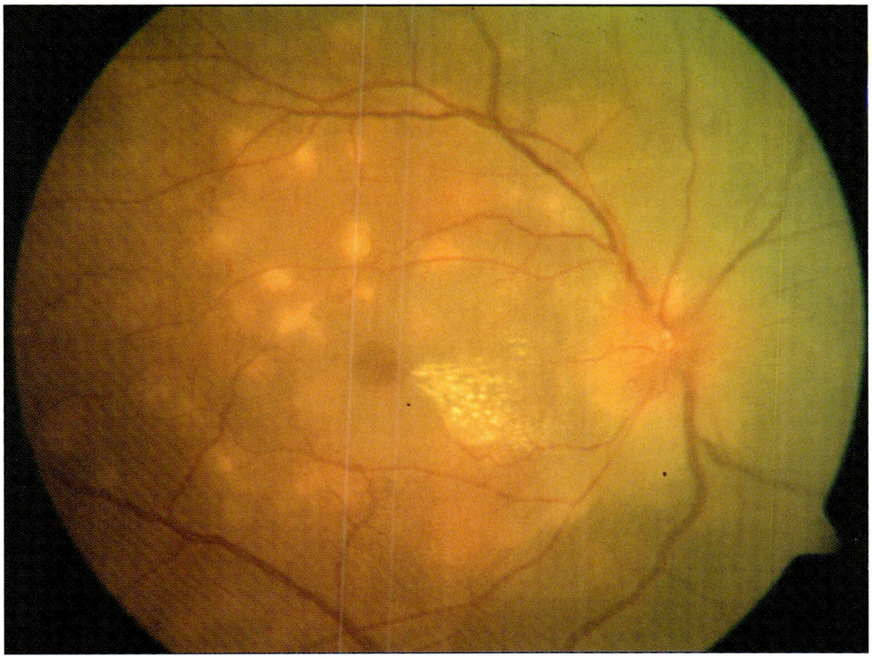

Choroiditis is a chorioretinal inflammatory disease of unknown etiology associated with vitritis and anterior uveitis. It affects young healthy adults usually in the third decade and more commonly in women. There is no known systemic disease association. It can present as focal, multifocal and disseminated choroiditis.

- Focal—Toxocariasis, tuberculosis, lymphoma
- Multifocal—Sarcoidosis, symphathetic ophthalmia, miliary tuberculosis, punctate inner choroidopathy
- Disseminated—Tuberculosis, serpiginous choroiditis.

Ocular Features

Symptoms

Blurred vision, scotoma, floaters, photopsia.

Signs

- Usually bilateral, mild to moderate anterior uveitis
- Fundus reveals multiple round or oval, yellow gray lesions (50-350 μm) at the level of RPE throughout posterior pole and mid periphery.
- Optic disc hyperemia and macular edema may occur.
- Healed lesions show round punched out scars with varying degree of hyperpigmentation.

Complications

Choroidal neovascular membrane, subretinal fibrosis, peripapillary atrophy

Investigations

- Fluorescein angiography: Active lesions show early hypofluorescence with late staining and leakage. Atrophic scars show early and late hyperfluorescence
- Indocyanine green angiography: Shows areas of hypofluorescence indicative of foci of active choroidal inflammation.

Treatment

- Corticosteroids (oral, periocular)
- Immunosuppressives

REFERENCES

1. Bhende PS, Biswas J, Madhavan HN: Serological evidence for active Epstein-Barr virus infection in multifocal choroiditis. Ind J Pathol Microbiol 1997;40:129-131.
2. Quillen DA, Davis JB, Gottlieb JL, Blodi BA, Callanan DG, Chang TS, Equi RA. The white dot syndromes. Am J Ophthalmol 2004;137:538-550.

Focal Choroiditis

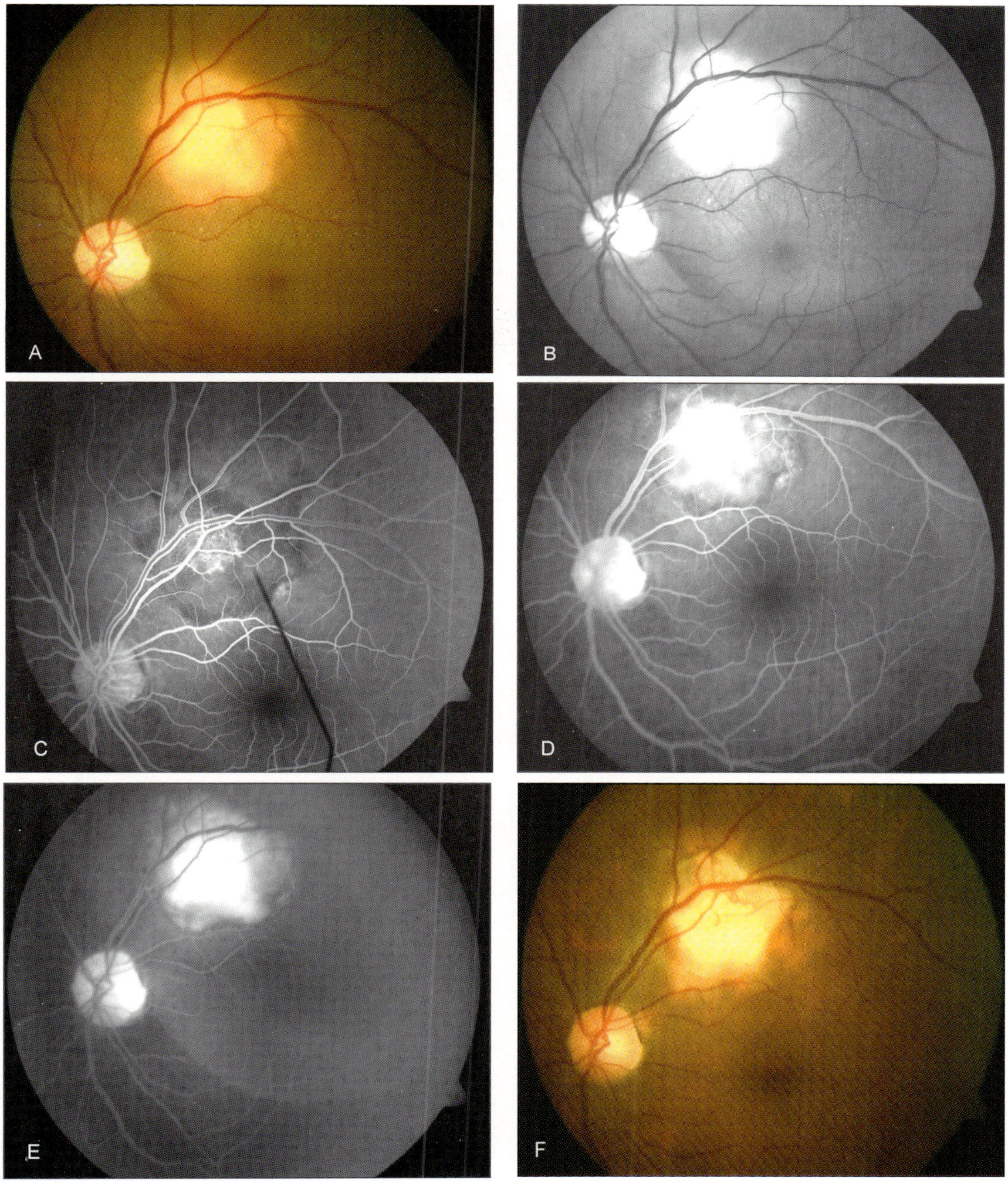

Figs. 13.1A to F:

A. Fundus photograph of a 36-year-old patient showing an active focus of tuberculous choroiditis along the superotemporal arcade along with subretinal fluid involving the macula

B. Red free photo of the same eye corresponding to the clinical picture

C-E Fluorescein angiogram showed early hypofluorescence followed by hyperfluorescence and staining of the lesion in the late phase

F. Fundus photograph showed regressed lesion in the choroid following antitubercular therapy. Laboratory investigations revealed raised ESR and a positive Mantoux test. The patient had enlarged cervical and supraclavicular lymph nodes

Acute Multifocal Choroiditis

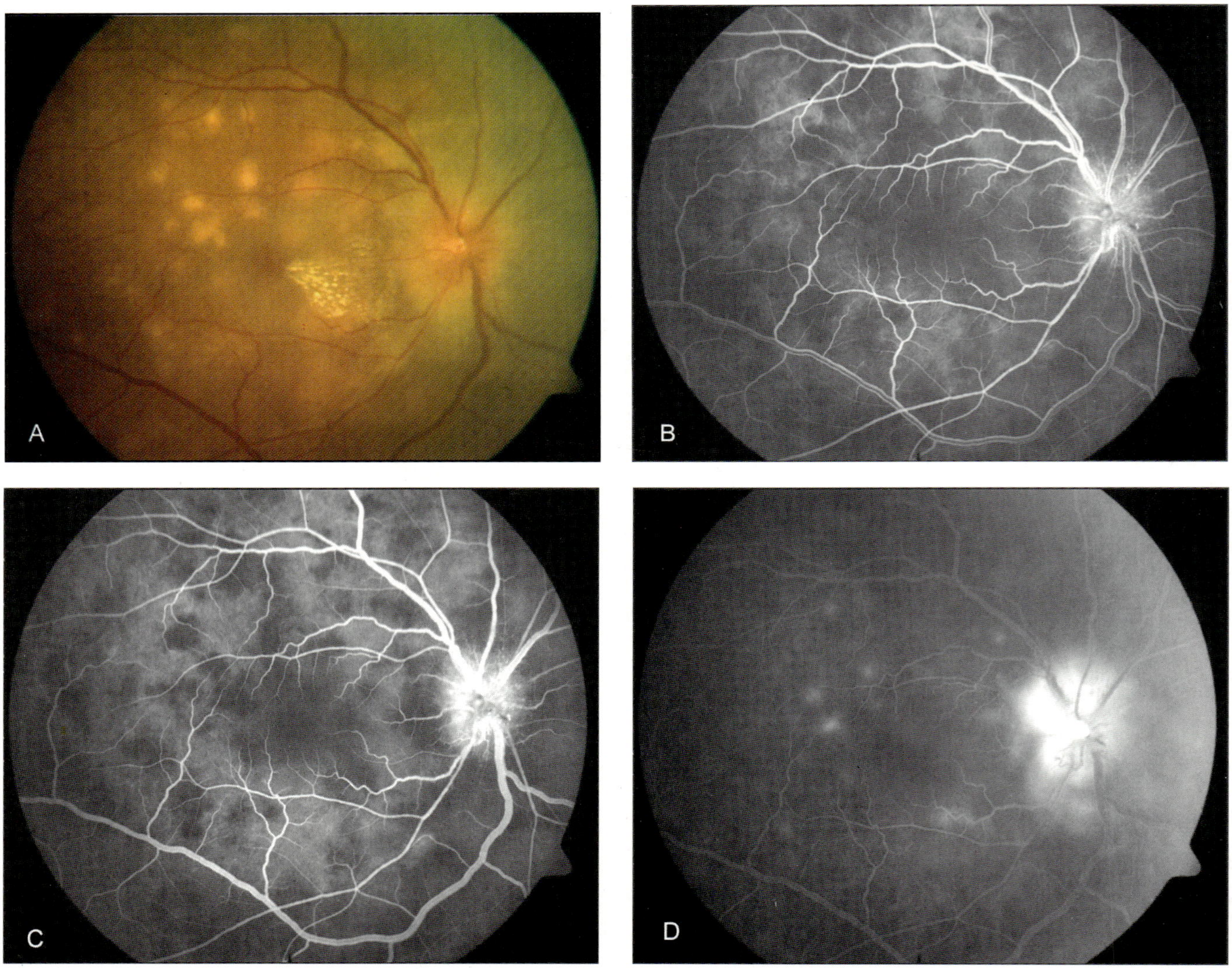

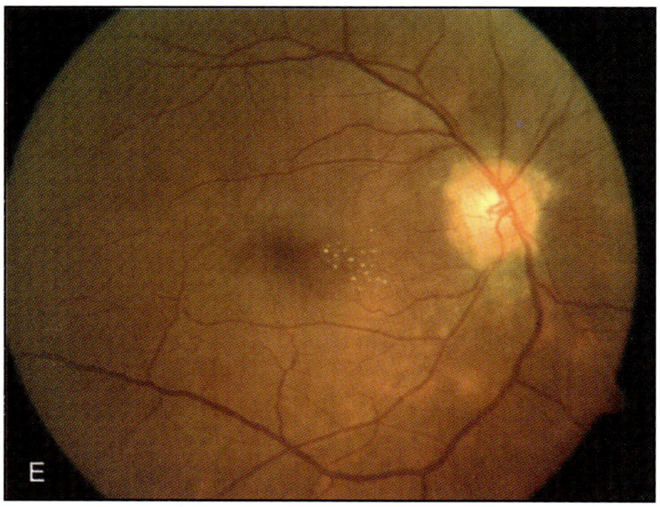

Figs 13.2A to E: A 45-year-old female complained of sudden diminution of vision in her right eye for a week.

A. Fundus photograph revealed multiple yellow round to oval sub retinal lesions in the posterior pole, few hard exudates along with disc edema

B-D Fluorescein angiogram showed early hypofluorescence with late staining of the lesions and the disc

E. Resolution of lesions following a course of systemic steroids and immunosuppressives.

Complications of Multifocal Choroiditis

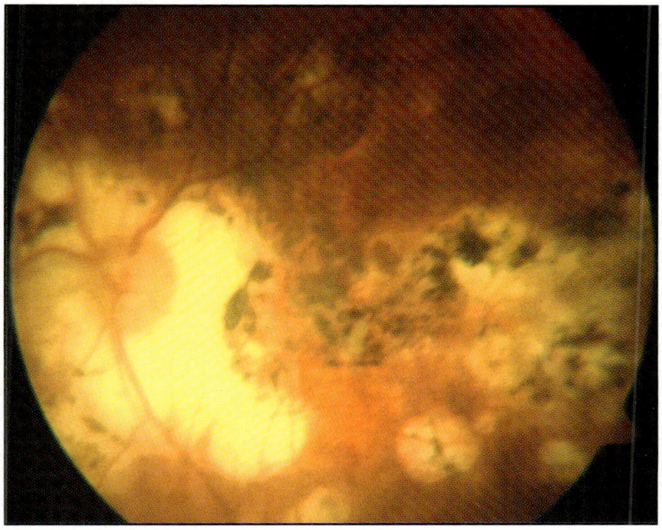

Fig. 13.3: Fundus photograph of healed disseminated choroiditis with extensive subretinal scarring and pigmentary changes over the macula.

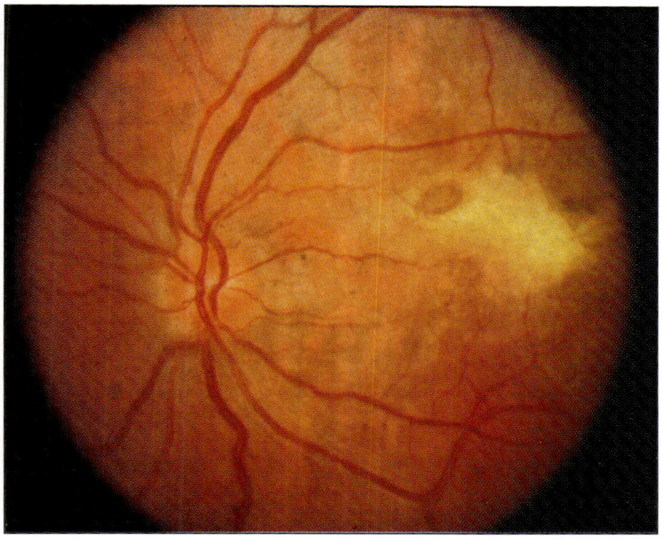

Fig. 13.4: Fundus photograph of subretinal fibrosis in a case of choroiditis

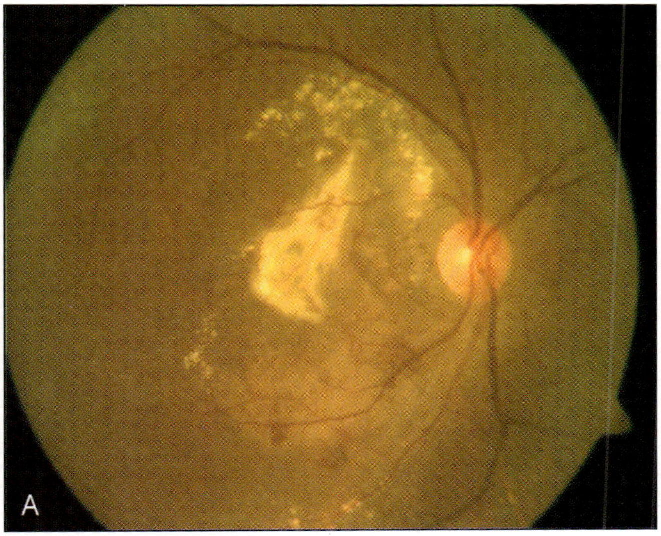

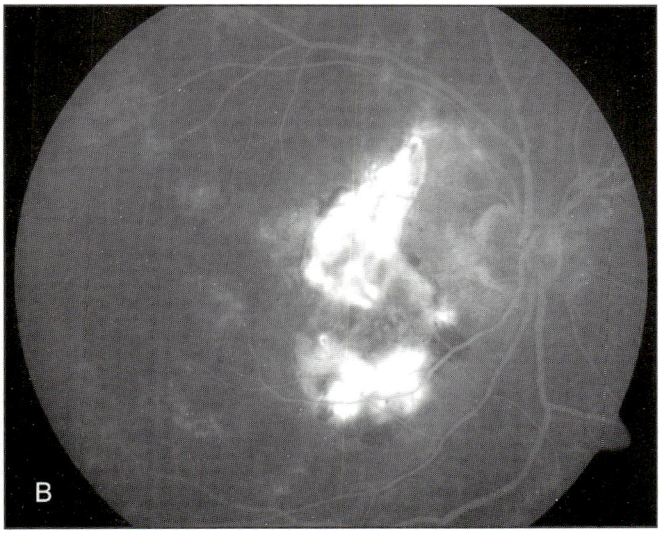

Figs 13.5A and B:
A. Fundus photograph of the right eye of a patient with multifocal choroiditis complicated by choroidal neovascular membrane
B. Fluorescein angiogram of the same eye showing staining of the lesion in the late phase

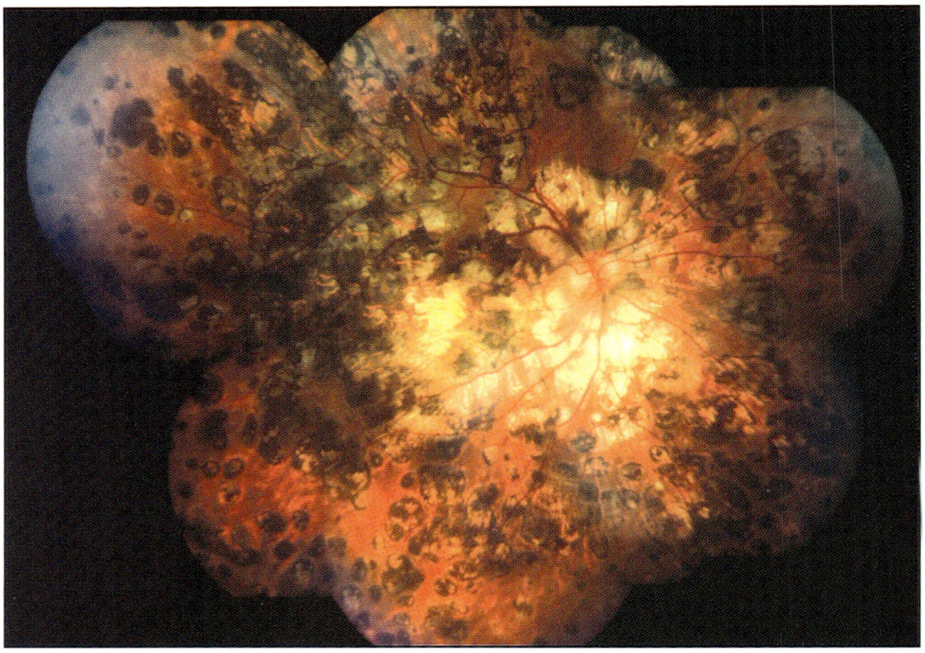

Fig. 13.6: Fundus photograph shows healed disseminated choroiditis

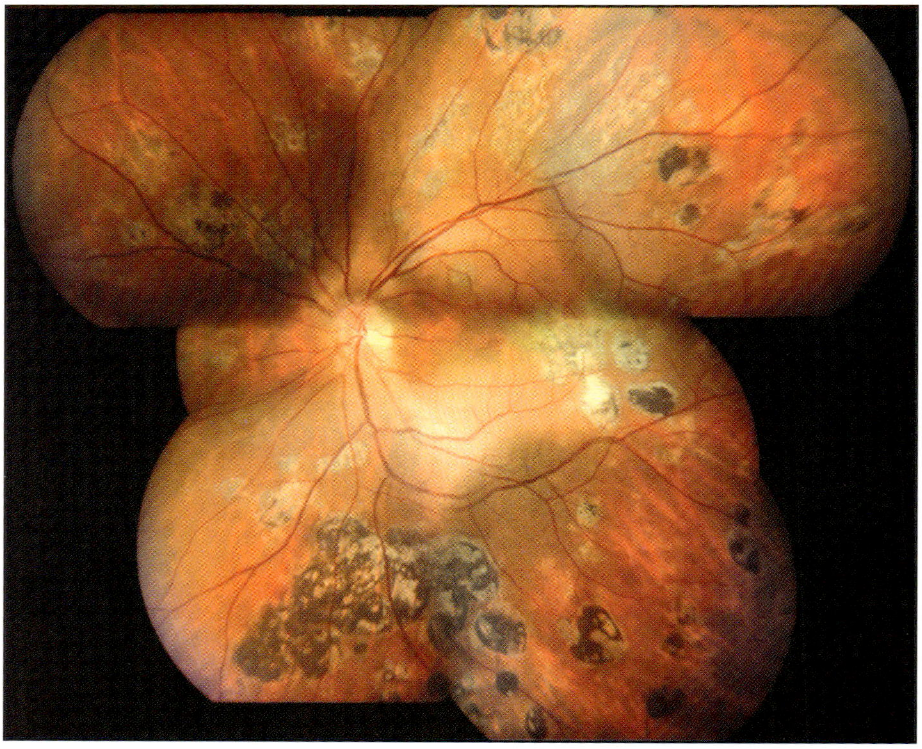

Fig. 13.7: Fundus photograph shows areas of healed choroiditis with pigmentary alterations

CHAPTER FOURTEEN

Ocular Toxoplasmosis

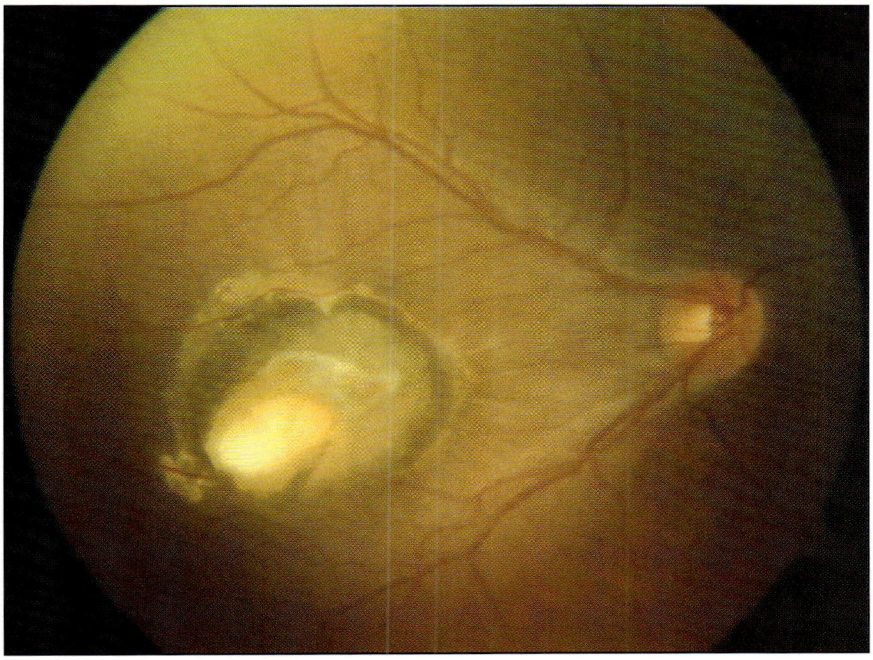

Toxoplasmosis is the most common cause of infectious retinochoroiditis in humans. It is caused by *Toxoplasma gondii,* an obligate intracellular protozoan parasite. Cat is the only definitive host. Human is the intermediate host. *T. gondii* exists in three forms:

1. Oocyst—soil form
2. Tachyzoite—active infectious form
3. Tissue cyst/bradyzoite—latent form

Human infection is either congenital or acquired by ingestion of the raw or undercooked meat, contaminated fruits,vegetables, drinking water or unpasteurized milk.

Ocular Features

Ocular toxoplasmosis causes 30-50 percent cases of posterior uveitis.

Symptoms

Children: Decreased vision, nystagmus, strabismus.

Adults: Blurred vision, floaters.

Signs

Dense vitritis, yellowish white focal retinitis adjacent to a pigmented chorioretinal scar, vasculitis, papillitis, neuroretinitis, optic neuritis.

In immunosuppressed patients, lesions may be bilateral, multifocal and atypical.

Complications

Choroidal neovascular membrane, optic atrophy, rhegmatogenous retinal detachment.

Investigations

- ELISA (serum and aqueous), Antitoxoplasma IgG and IgM antibodies
- Polymerase chain reaction (PCR) of aqueous aspirate CT /MRI Brain in cases of toxoplasmic encephalitis especially in immunosuppressed patients.

Treatment

- Antitoxoplasmic drugs—Pyrimethamine, sulphadiazine, clindamycin, azithromycin, trimethoprim + sulphamethoxazole, atovaquone. Spiramycin is the drug of choice in pregnancy.
- Corticosteroids

REFERENCES

1. Holland GN, Lewis KG. An update on current practices in the management of ocular toxoplasmosis. Am J Ophthalmol 2002; 134:102-114.
2. Stanford MR, Sarah E. See, Leanne V. Jones, and Gilbert RE. Antibiotics for toxoplasmic retinochoroiditis: An evidence-based systematic review. Ophthalmology 2003;110: 926-932.
3. Holland GN. Ocular toxoplasmosis: A global reassessment: epidemiology and course of disease.Am J Ophthalmol 2003; 136:973-988.
4. Holland GN. Ocular toxoplasmosis: A global reassessment: Disease manifestations and management.Am J Ophthalmol 2004; 137:1-17.

Ocular Features of Toxoplasmosis

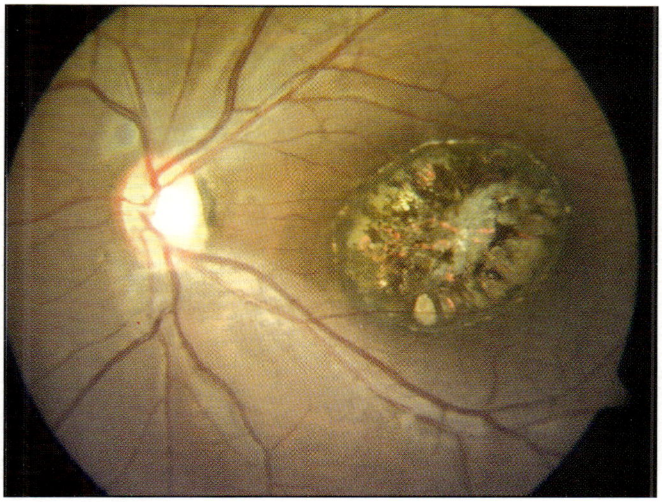

Fig. 14.1: Congenital toxoplasmic retinochoroidal scar

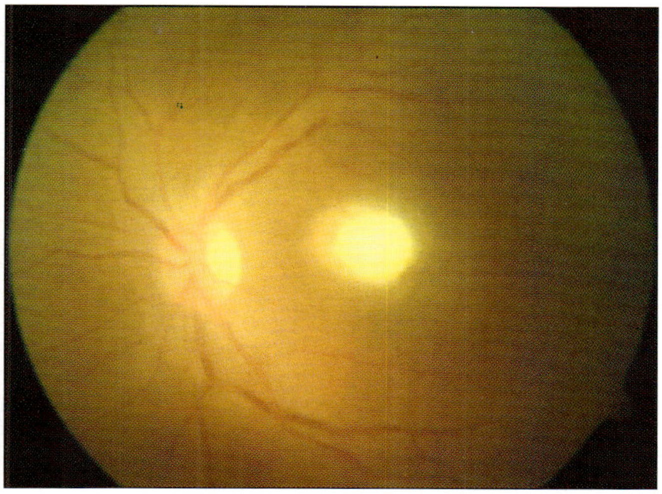

Fig. 14.2: Acquired active toxoplasmic retinochoroiditis in a 35-year-old lady who gave a history of contact with pet cats and dogs. There were no previous scars

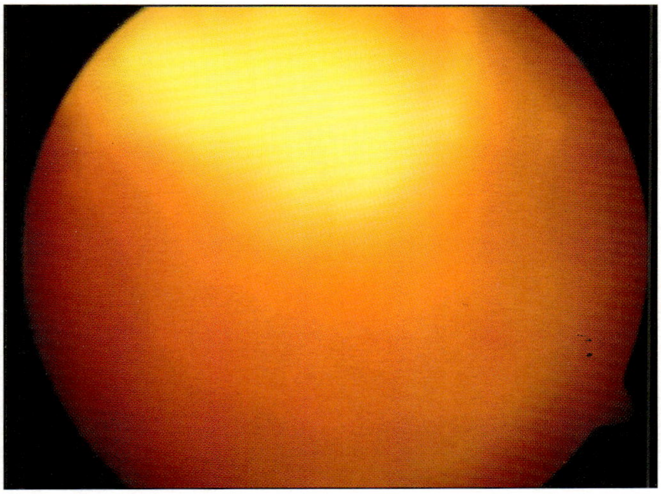

Fig. 14.3: Active toxoplasma retinitis with severe vitritis giving rise to 'headlight in the fog' appearance

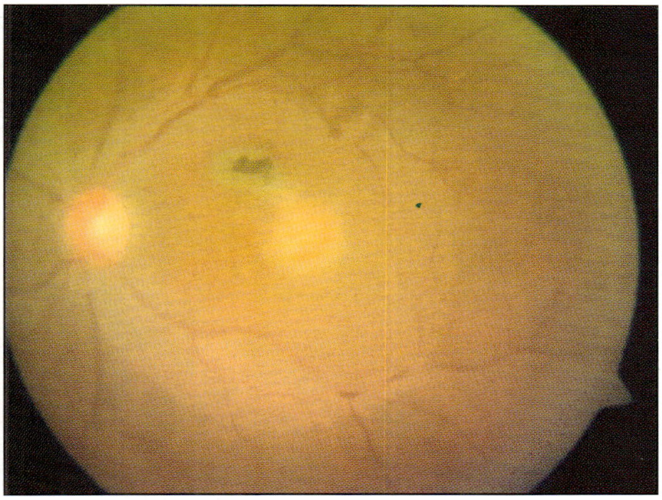

Fig. 14.4: Reactivation of toxoplasmic retinochoroiditis in the foveal region adjacent to an old toxoplasmic retinochoroidal scar

Acquired Focal Toxoplasmic Retinochoroiditis

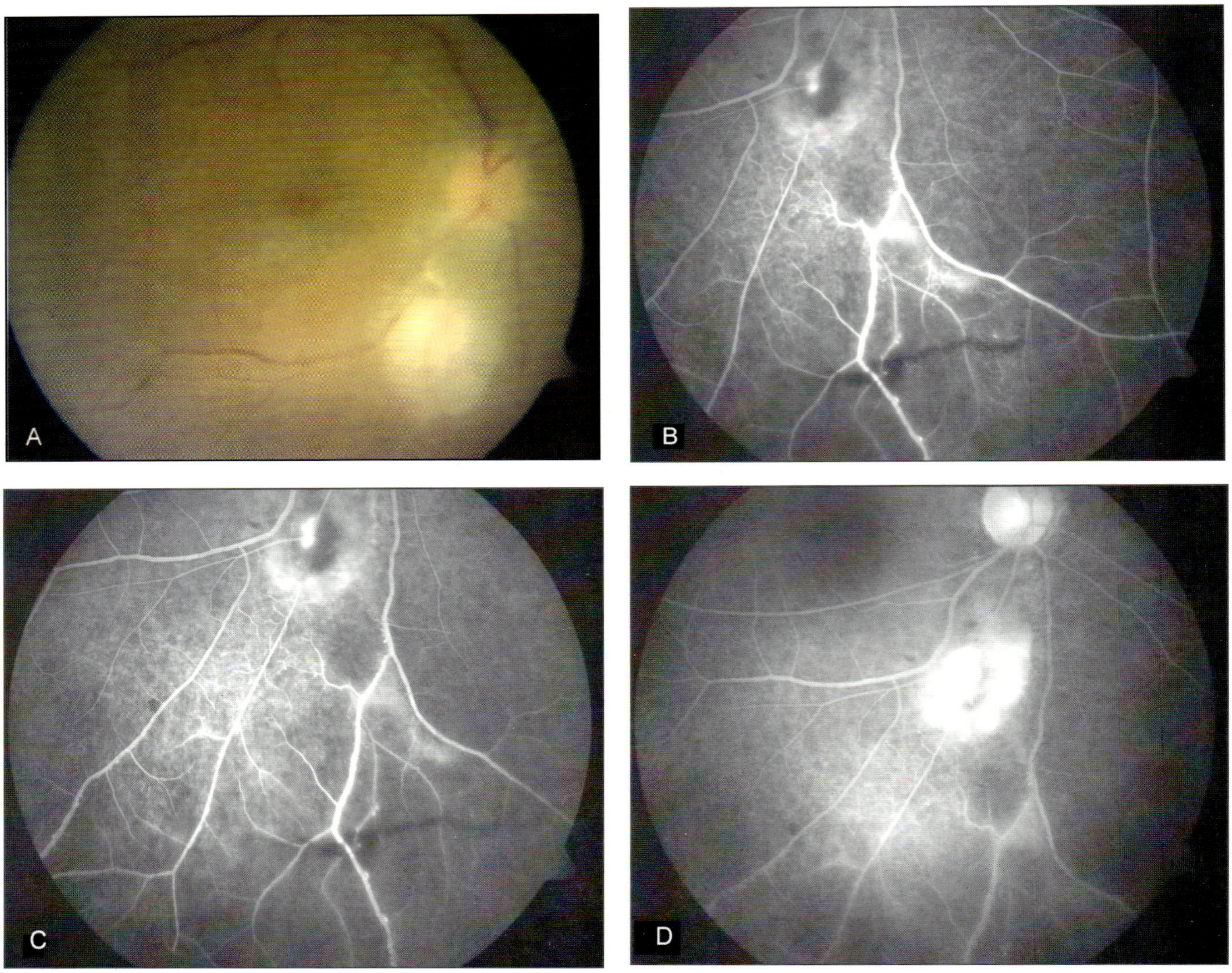

Figs 14.5A to D: (A) Acquired focal toxoplasmic retinochoroiditis along the inferotemporal arcade in the right eye associated with phlebitis. ELISA titers for IgG and IgM toxoplasma were raised. (B to D) Fluorescein angiogram showed blocked fluorescence due to active lesion and surrounding retinal edema in the early phase. Few areas of capillary nonperfusion were also seen due to occlusive vasculitis. Late phase showed hyperfluorescence corresponding to the active lesions

Reactivation of an Old Toxoplasmic Scar

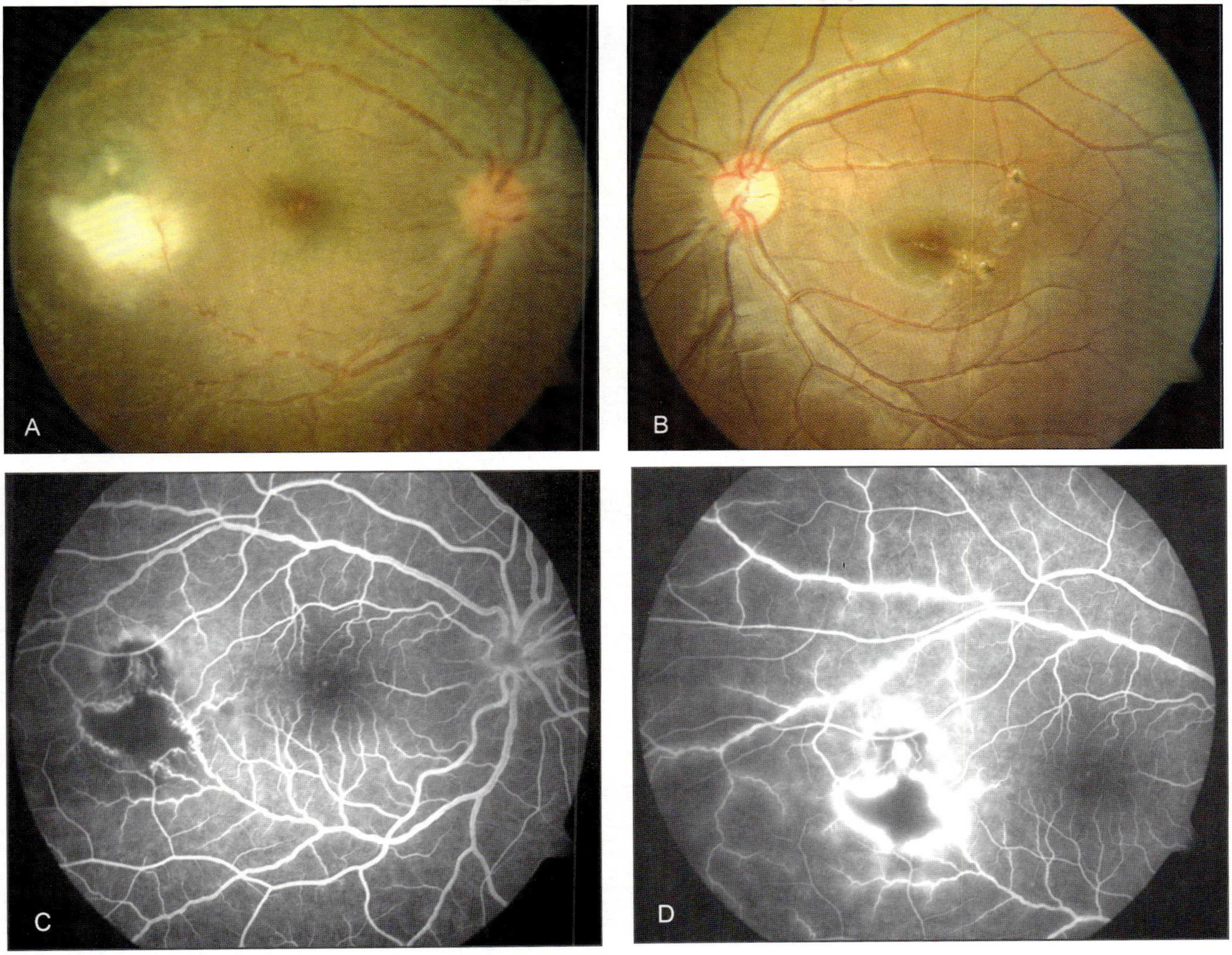

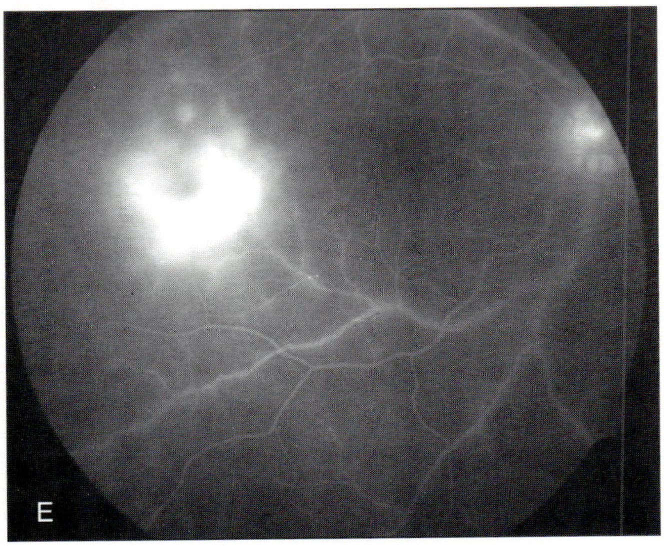

Figs 14.6A to E: (A) Active toxoplasma retinochoroiditis adjacent to an old pigmented scar along with surrounding retinal edema and periphlebitis in the right eye of a patient. (B) Left eye of the same patient showing pigmented chorioretinal scars in the posterior pole. (C to E) Fundus fluorescein angiogram shows early blocked fluorescence due to retinal inflammation followed by active leakage at the site of lesion and inflamed vessels in the late phase

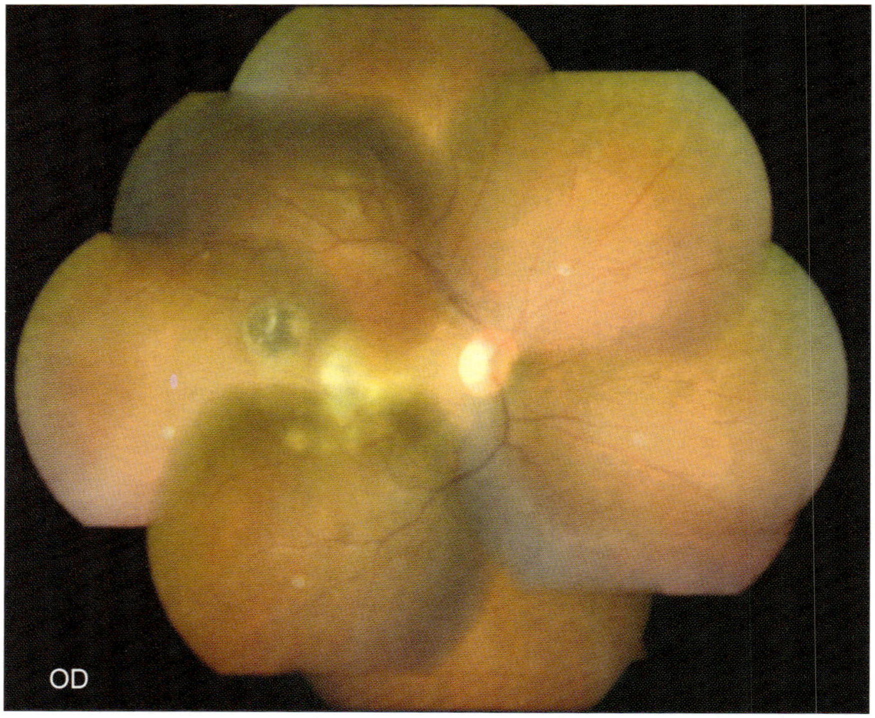

Fig. 14.7: A focus of recurrent toxoplasmic retinochoroidal lesion adjacent to an old scar in the macular area. Antitoxoplasma treatment along with systemic steroids was given following which lesion resolved

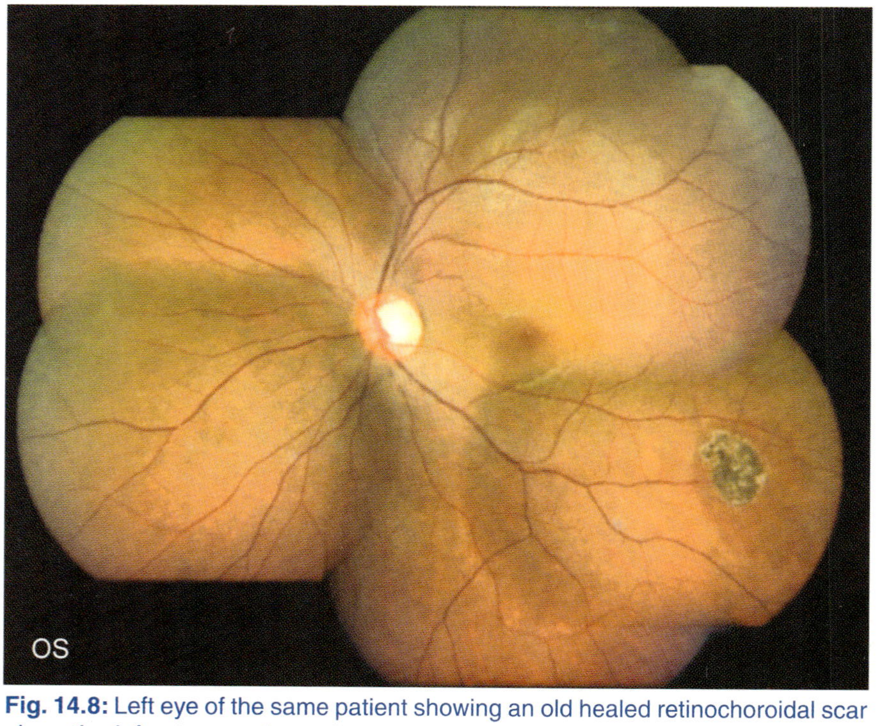

Fig. 14.8: Left eye of the same patient showing an old healed retinochoroidal scar along the inferotemporal arcade

Complications of Toxoplasmic Retinochoroiditis

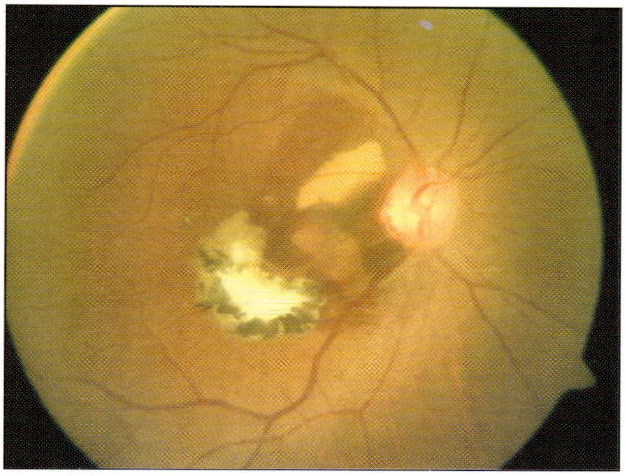

Fig. 14.9: Fundus photograph shows choroidal neovascular membrane adjacent to a toxoplasmic scar

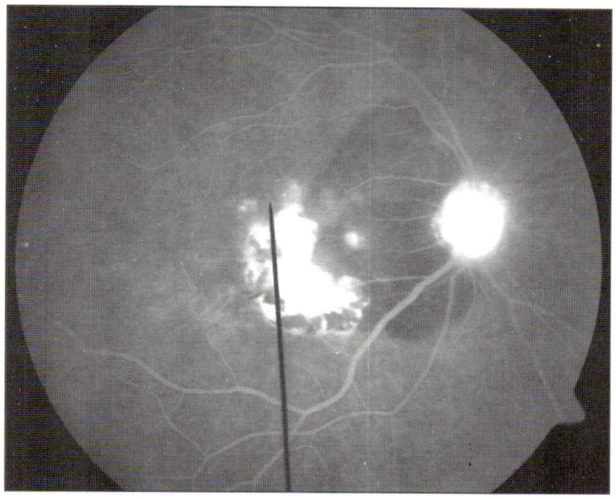

Fig. 14.10: Fluorescein angiogram shows blocked fluorescence corresponding to the hemorrhage and a hyperfluorescence consistent with neovascular membrane

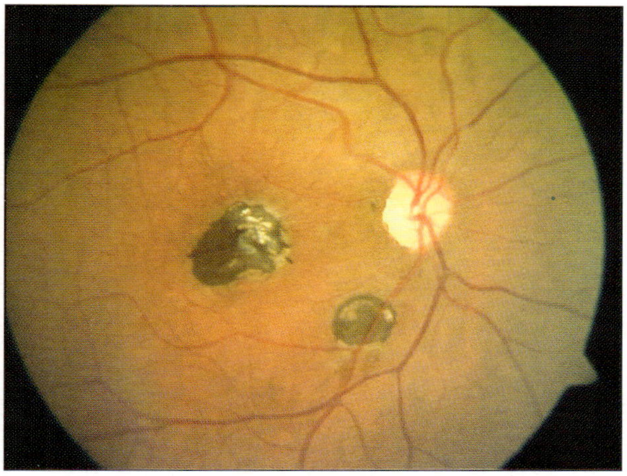

Fig. 14.11: Clinical photograph showing pigment clumping in chorioretinal scar following toxoplasma infection

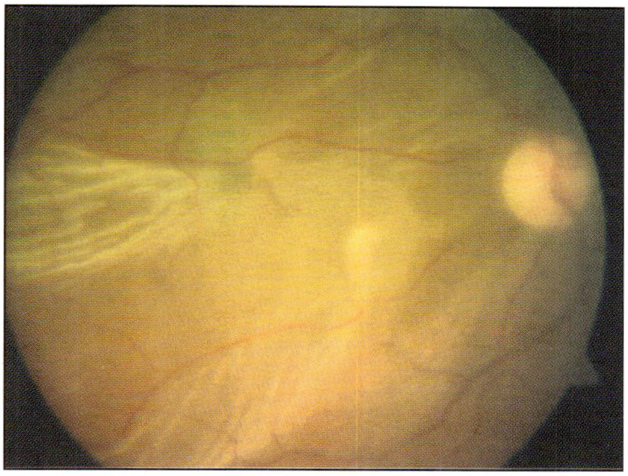

Fig. 14.12: Rhegmatogenous retinal detachment in a patient with toxoplasmic retinochoroiditis following 2 months of antitoxo treatment. The retinal break was located next to the chorioretinal atrophic patch

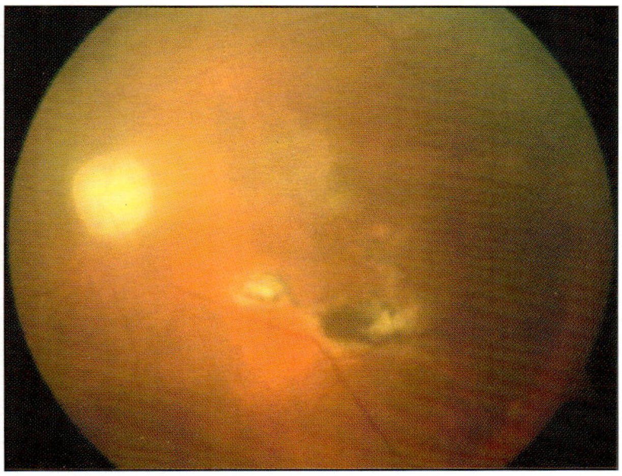

Fig. 14.13: Optic disc pallor in a patient with toxoplasmic retinochoroiditis

Atypical Presentations of Toxoplasmic Retinochoroiditis

Toxoplasmosis in AIDS

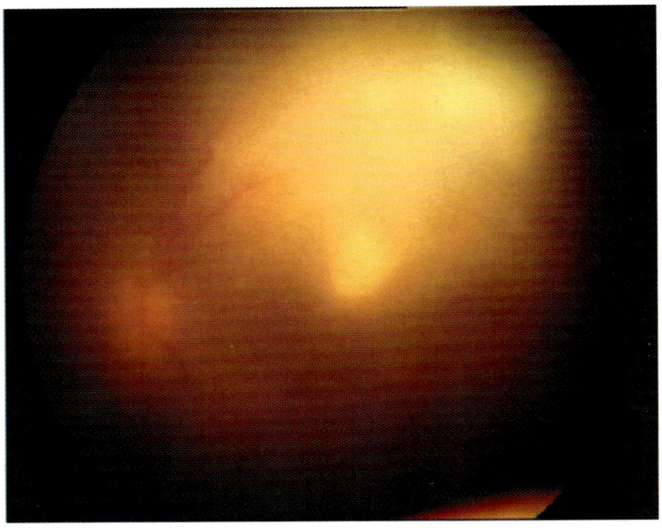

Fig. 14.14: Multifocal toxoplasmic retinochoroiditis in an AIDS patient

Frosted branch angiitis in a patient with toxoplasmosis

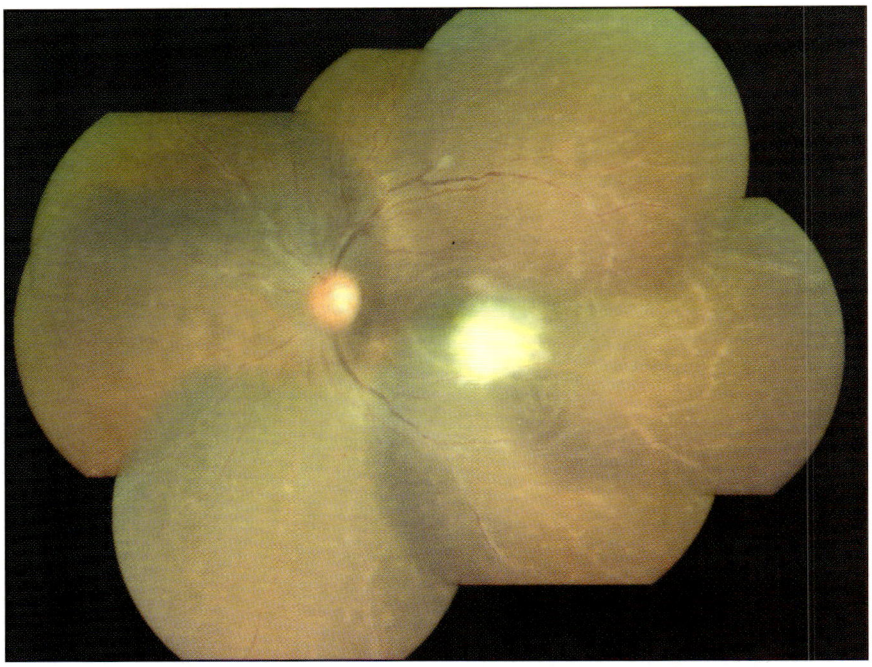

Fig. 14.15: A 13-year-old boy came in our clinic with complaints of decreased vision for 10 days. Fundus examination showed active retinochoroidal lesion in the foveal region along with frosted branch angiitis. Aqueous and serum sample showed high titers of IgG and IgM for *Toxoplasma gondii*. The patient was treated with antitoxotherapy for a period of 2 months following which retinitis resolved

CHAPTER FIFTEEN

Parasitic Uveitis

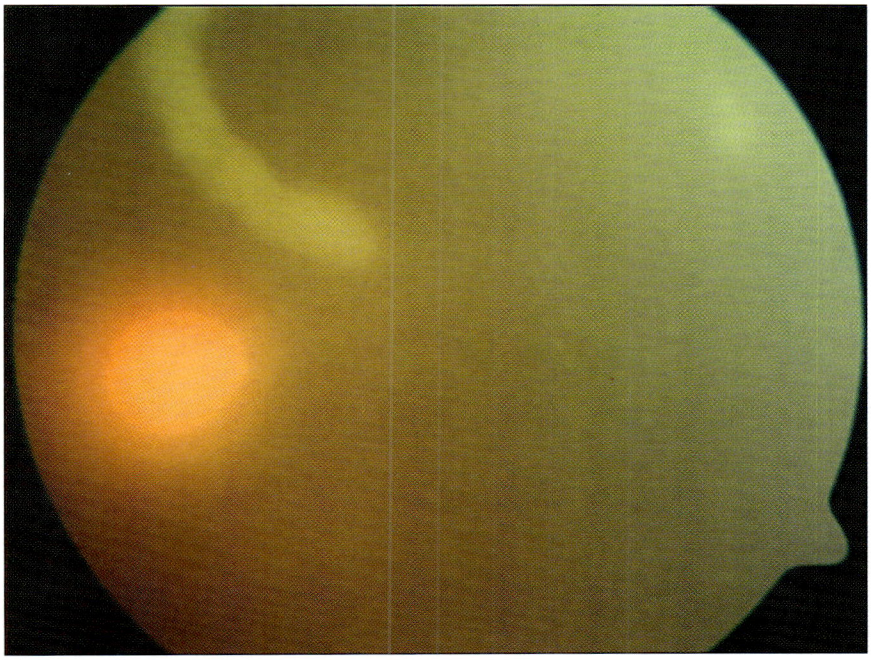

TOXOCARIASIS

It is a zoonotic disease caused by the infestation of humans by the second stage larvae of the dog nematode Toxocara canis or the cat nematode T. cati.Human beings are infected through ingestion of the ova from contaminated food or by close contact with puppies.

Ocular Features (Ocular larva migrans)

A. Peripheral granuloma seen as an elevated white mass typically associated with retinal folds extending towards the granuloma.
B. Posterior pole granuloma which is white or gray, round and elevated, usually 1-2 disc diameters in size and centered in the juxta papillary or subfoveal location.
C. Chronic endophthalmitis is usually associated with retinal detachment, mild anterior uveitis, posterior synechiae and a cyclitic membrane between the detached retina and the lens.

Systemic Clinical Manifestations (Visceral larva migrans)

It is seen in young children (3 to 5 years of age) with a history of pica. Symptoms include fever, nausea, coughing, wheezing, weight loss, hepatomegaly and pruritic eruptions over the body.

Investigations

ELISA for anti toxocara antibody.

Treatment

- Asymptomatic seropositive individuals/Quiescent ocular disease – No therapy
- Visceral larva migrans – Anti-inflammatory agents with antihelminthic agents
- Ocular toxocariasis – Systemic or periocular steroids with concomitant antihelminthic agents. Posterior vitrectomy may also be needed to remove inflammatory tissues, relieve vitreous traction, reduce retinal distortion and repair tractional – rhegmatogenous detachment.

REFERENCE

1. Sabrosa NA, Zajdenweber M. Nematode infections of the eye: toxocariasis, onchocerciasis, diffuse unilateral subacute neuroretinitis, and cysticercosis. Ophthalmol Clin North Am. 2002; 15(3): 351-6.

Toxocariasis

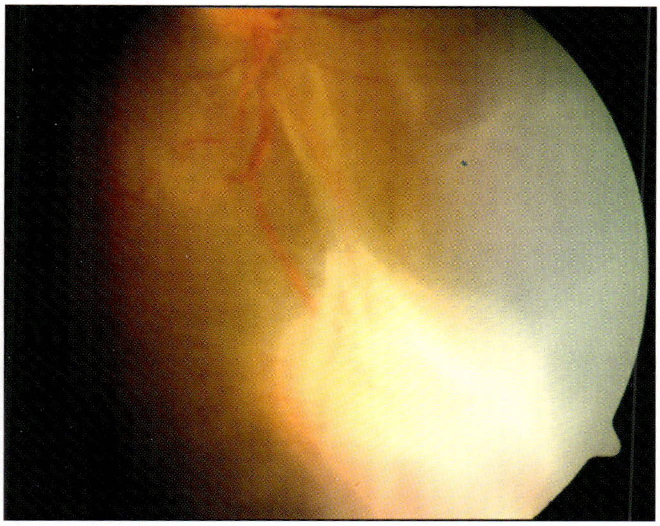

Fig. 15.1: Fundus photograph showing peripheral toxocara granuloma with traction bands extending from the disc to the granuloma

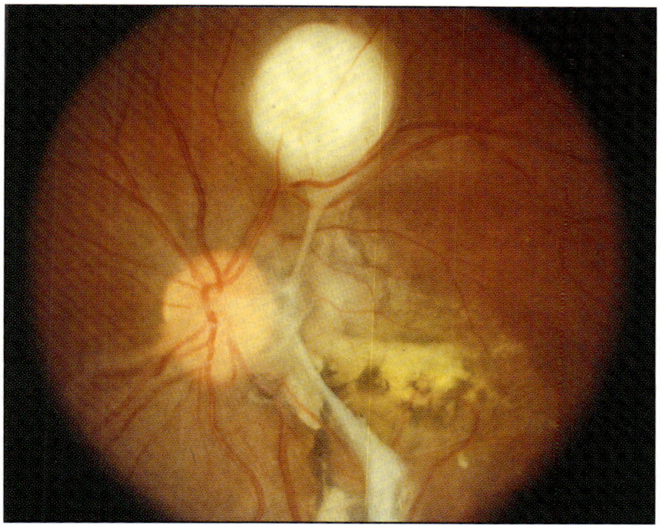

Fig. 15.2: A quiescent toxocara granuloma in the posterior pole with fibrotic bands involving disc and macula

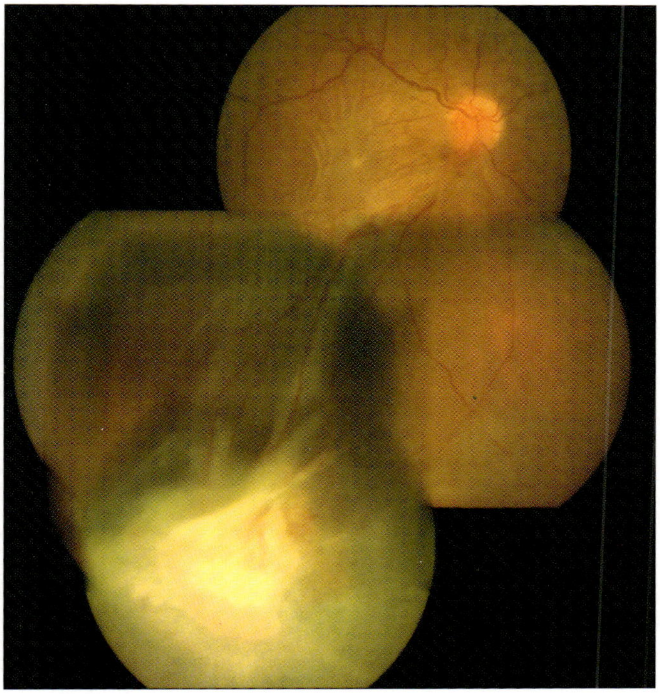

Fig. 15.3: Montage photograph showing peripheral toxocara granuloma inferiorly causing straightening of retinal vessels and tractional retinal detachment

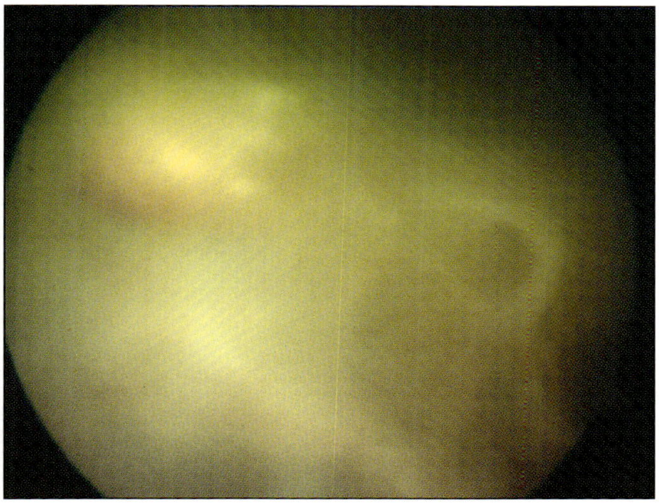

Fig. 15.4: Fundus photograph showing toxocara granuloma in the periphery with dense vitreitis

DIFFUSE UNILATERAL SUBACUTE NEURORETINOPATHY

Gass et al first described it in 1978. The causative organisms are *Ankylostoma caninum* and *Baylisascaris procyonis*. It usually affects healthy young patients with no preceding illness and no past ocular history.

Ocular Features

Early Stage

Symptoms: Unilateral paracentral or central scotoma, ocular discomfort or transient visual obscurations.

Signs: Mild anterior segment inflammation, vitreitis, papillitis, and multiple gray-white lesions in the deep retina with scattered areas of depigmentation. A motile subretinal worm may also be seen on indirect ophthalmoscopy.

Late Stage

Symptoms: Profound visual loss with dense central and patchy peripheral visual field loss.

Signs: Disc pallor, retinal arteriole narrowing, areas of RPE atrophy

Investigations

A. Complete blood count , specially eosinophil counts
B. Stool examination—ova and parasites
C. ELISA—Toxocara canis , Baylisascaris procyonis.
D. ERG—loss of "B" wave with relative preservation of "a" wave ; ERG rarely extinguished even in late stages

Treatment

Argon laser photocoagulation is the only effective way to eliminate the worm without any known severe reaction. Chemotherapy with antihelminthic drug, *thiabendazole* along with steroids may help when the worm cannot be visualized.

REFERENCES

1. Gass JD, Gilbert WR Jr, Guerry R, et al. Diffuse unilateral subacute neuroretinitis. Ophthalmology 1978;85:521.
2. Mets MB, Noble AG, Basti S, Gavin P, Davis AT, Shulman ST, Kazacos KR. Eye findings of diffuse unilateral subacute neuroretinitis and multiple choroidal infiltrates associated with neural larva migrans due to Baylisascaris procyonis. Am J Ophthalmol. 2003;135:888-90.

Diffuse Unilateral Subacute Neuroretinitis (DUSN)

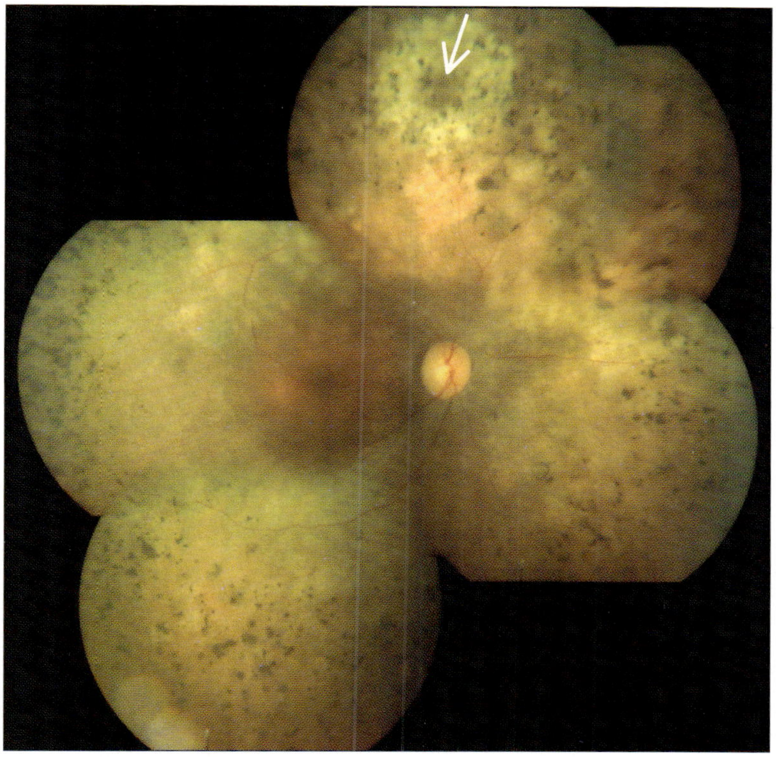

Fig. 15.5: Montage fundus photograph showing diffuse unilateral subacute neuroretinitis in a patient with retinitis pigmentosa like fundus appearance. Diffuse yellow-white deep retinal lesions were seen scattered throughout the fundus. Superiorly, a subretinal motile worm was seen around which laser photocoagulation (arrow) was done

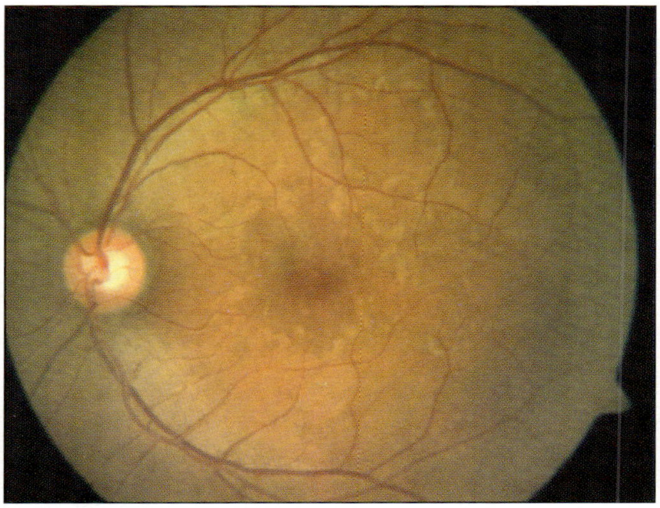

Fig. 15.6: Fundus photograph of a patient showing multiple RPE tracts caused by ocular larvae migrans

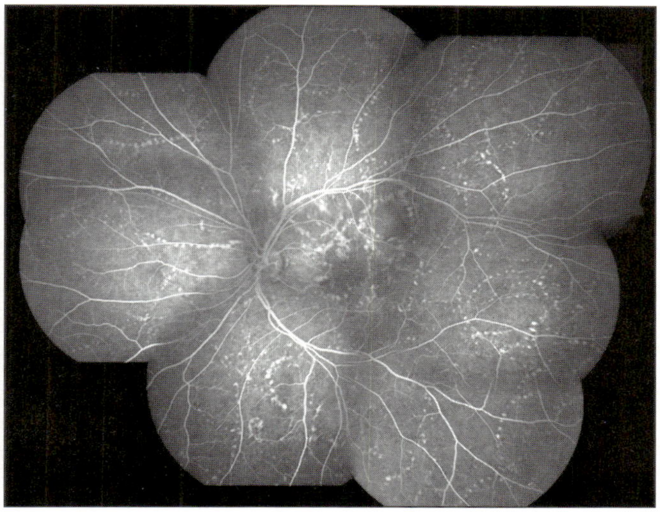

Fig. 15.7: Fluorescein angiogram of the same eye showing multiple linear hyperfluorescent lesions suggestive of RPE tracts of DUSN

FILARIASIS

Threadlike adult worms in subcutaneous tissues and lymphatics reproduce sexually to produce microfilariae, causing a range of manifestations.

Dirofilariasis

- D. immitis—heartworm of dogs, D. repens—cats and dogs, D. tenuis—raccoons.
- Vectors—Culex and Aedes; accidental transmission to humans
- Ophthalmic infections –
  a. Eyelids, periorbital tissues, orbit
  b. Conjunctiva, anterior chamber, vitreous
- Most common clinical presentation is "well-encapsulated nonviable parasite"

Diagnosis—ELISA test.

Treatment—Surgical removal.

Lymphatic Filariasis

- Propensity for lymphatic migration—*Wuchereria bancrofti, Brugia malayi, Brugia timori*
- Ocular filariasis is rare

REFERENCES

1. Sabrosa NA, Zajdenweber M. Nematode infections of the eye: toxocariasis, onchocerciasis, diffuse unilateral subacute neuroretinitis, and cysticercosis. Ophthalmol Clin North Am. 2002.
2. Ganesh SK, Babu K, Krishnakumar S, Biswas J. Ocular filariasis due to Wuchereria bancrofti presenting as panuveitis: A case report. Ocul Immunol Inflamm. 2003; 11: 145-148.

Ocular Filariasis

A 35-year-old lady complained of acute onset of pain, redness and photophobia in the right eye. Her best corrected vision was 20/60.

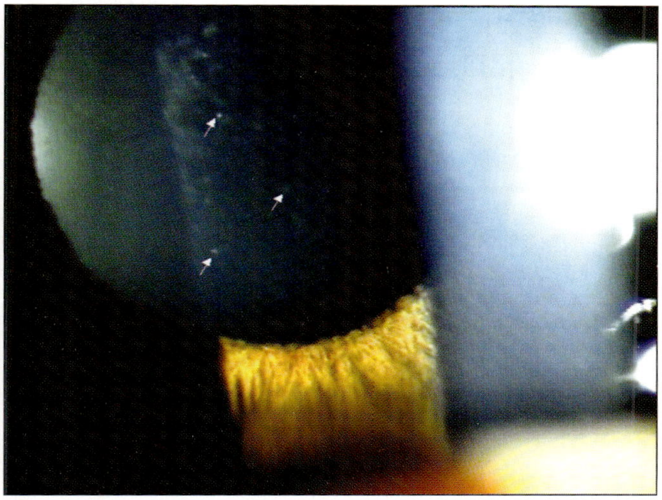

Fig. 15.8: Slit lamp photograph shows multiple, tiny, motile larvae in the anterior chamber

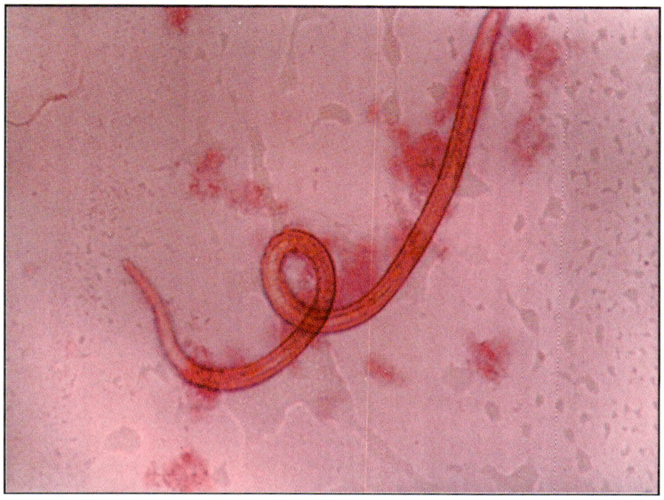

Fig. 15.9: Photomicrograph showing *Wuchereria bancrofti microfilariae* in peripheral blood smear

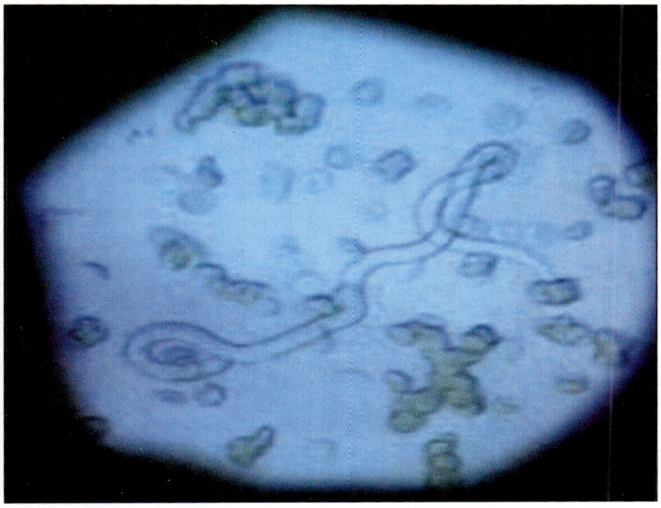

Fig. 15.10: Photomicrograph showing *Wuchereria bancrofti* microfilariae in aqueous tap

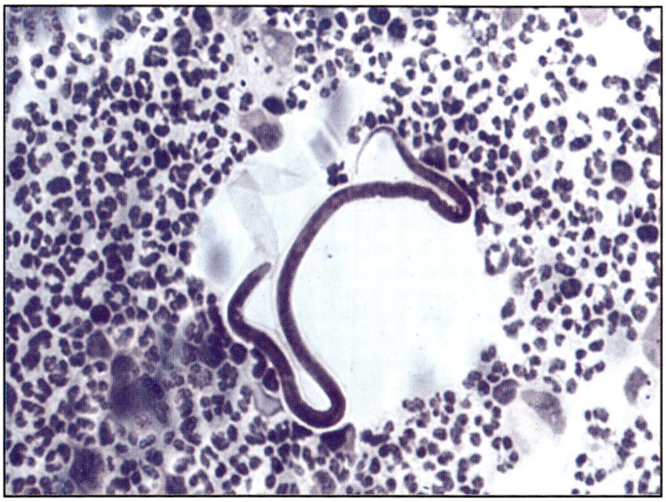

Fig. 15.11: Photomicrograph of anterior chamber aspirate showing *a microfilariae* surrounded by plenty of polymorphonuclear leucocytes and few macrophages in a patient who presented with anterior uveitis and hypopyon

CYSTICERCOSIS

Cysticercosis is the most common ocular tapeworm infection. It is caused by *Cysticercosis cellulosae* the larval form of pork tapeworm, *Taenia solium*. Humans become infected by drinking contaminated water or eating food containing the eggs of *Taenia solium*.

Ocular Features

Cysticercosis may affect any part of the eye, from orbit to visual cortex, however posterior segment involvement is the most common.

Symptoms—Decreased vision, floaters or flashes.

Signs—Vitritis, intravitreal or sub retinal cyst, and optic neuritis.

Diagnosis

- History of prior infection/travel to endemic areas
- Direct visualization as a translucent white cyst with a dense white spot (invaginated scolex) with a characteristic undulatory movement
- If media hazy, B–scan ultrasonography is useful.

Treatment

Medical treatment usually causes serious visual loss as degeneration of cyst incites severe inflammation. Surgical removal of the cyst is the treatment of choice.

REFERENCES

1. George AE, Biswas J, Agarwal R, Kumarasamy N, Solomon S. Subretinal cysticercosis in an AIDS patient – treatment with Xenon arc photocoagulation. Retina 1999; 19(5): 467-68.
2. Sabrosa NA, Zajdenweber M. Nematode infections of the eye: toxocariasis, onchocerciasis, diffuse unilateral subacute neuroretinitis, and cysticercosis. Ophthalmol Clin North Am 2002; 15: 351-56.
3. Sharma T, Sinha S, Shah N, Gopal L, Shanmugam MP, Bhende P, Bhende M, Shetty NS, Agrawal R, Deshpande D, Biswas J, Sukumar B. Intraocular cysticercosis: clinical characteristics and visual outcome after vitreoretinal surgery. Ophthalmology 2003;110 : 996-1004.

Cysticercosis

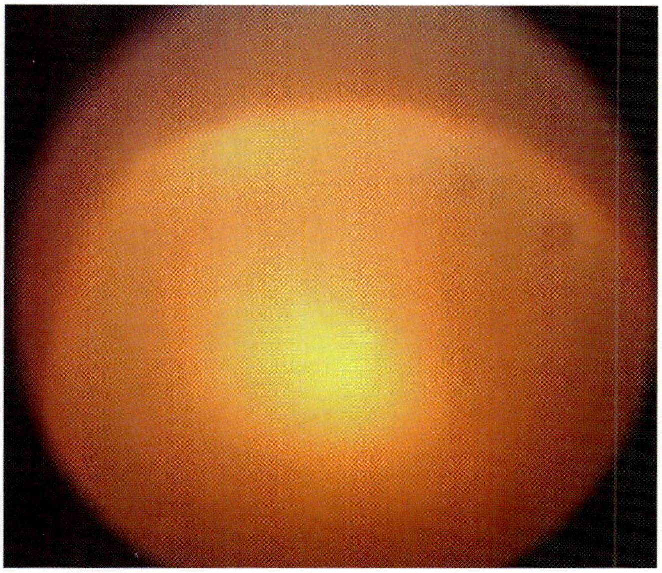

Fig. 15.12: Fundus photograph shows a cysticercosis cyst in the vitreous cavity

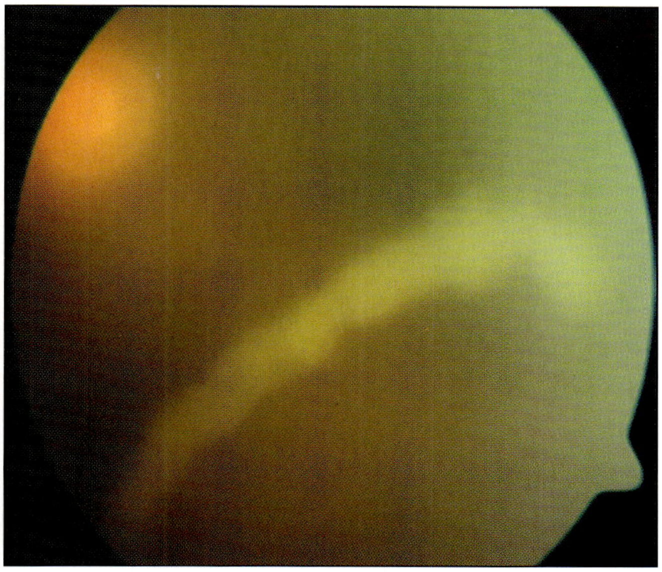

Fig. 15.13: Fundus photograph shows dense vitritis and a dead worm in the vitreous cavity

Gnathostomiasis

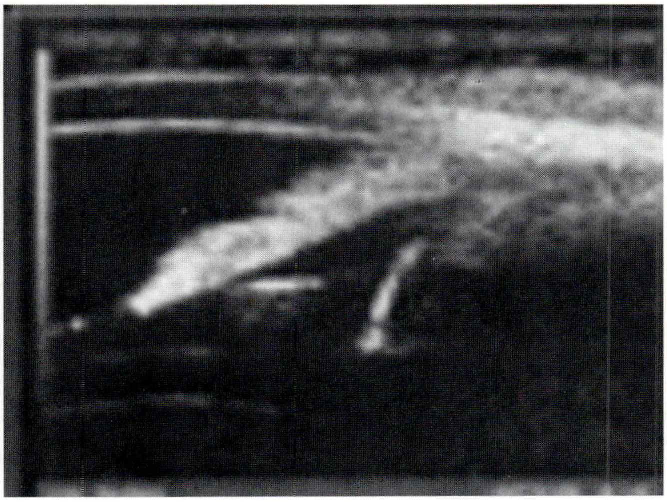

Fig. 15.14: Ultrasound biomicroscopy shows a high reflective echo extending from iris root into the posterior chamber suggestive of intraocular worm in the eye

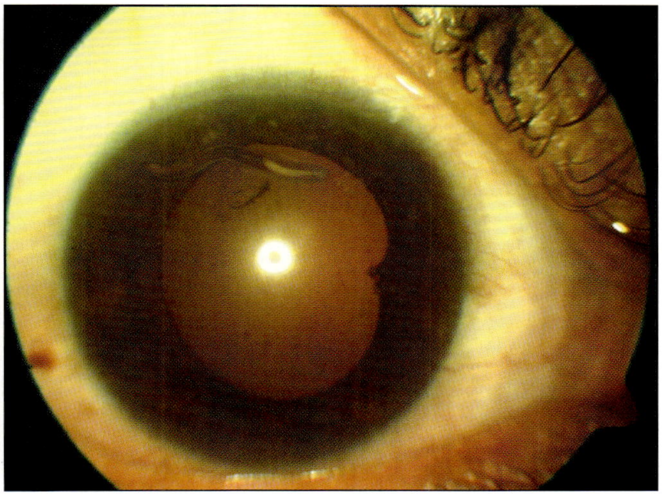

Fig. 15.15: Slit lamp photograph showing a dead intraocular worm stuck on the corneal endothelium and was diagnosed to be *Gnathostoma*

CHAPTER SIXTEEN

Viral Retinitis

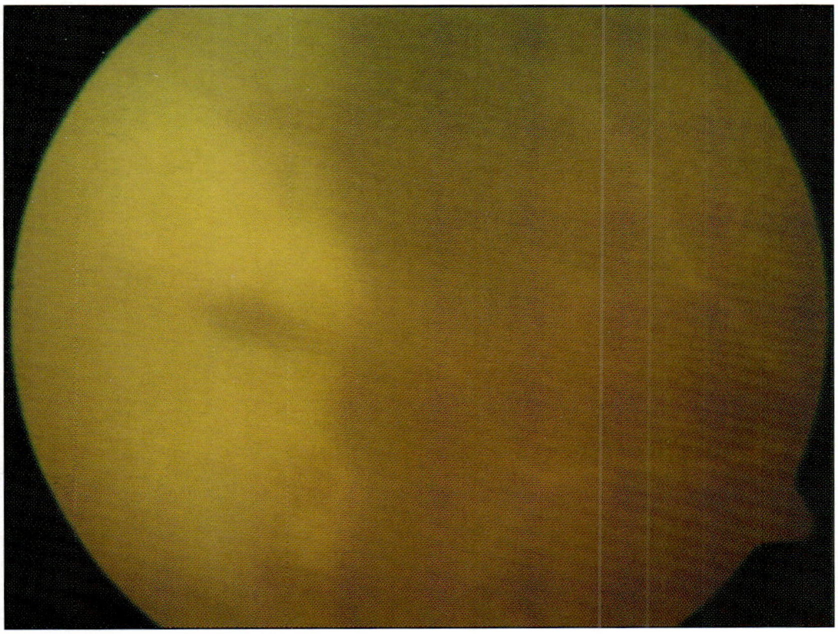

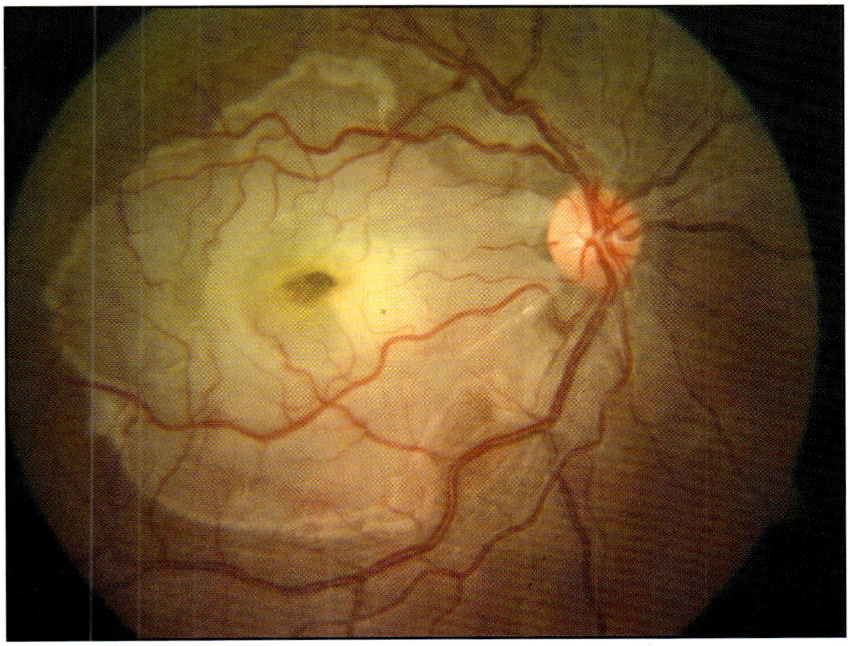

Intraocular inflammation by herpes group of viruses may manifest as either acute retinal necrosis (ARN) or necrotizing herpetic retinopathy caused by either herpes simplex virus or varicella zoster virus. The disease is more common in elderly, immunosuppressed patients, AIDS and malignancies.

Acute retinal necrosis is a fulminant, necrotizing viral infection of the retina. Urayama first described it in 1971. ARN occurs in healthy individuals of either age or sex. It may be bilateral in 33 percent of patients.

Ocular Features

Symptoms

Pain, redness, photophobia, blurred vision

Signs

- Anterior uveitis with keratic precipitates
- Necrotizing retinitis: The lesion starts as deep necrotizing yellow-white lesion at the periphery that later confluences concentrically. Deep "**thumbprint**" infiltrates may occur posterior to the equator, with isolated patches of necrotizing retinitis in the periphery. A sharp saw-toothed demarcation line separates necrotic from healthy retina. Vitreous haze and active vasculitis may also be present. Active retinitis lasts for 4-6 weeks following which pigmentation of peripheral lesion and retinal breaks occur.

Complications

Rhegmatogenous retinal detachment (50-75%), optic atrophy. The other eye may be involved in 33 percent of the cases.

Investigations

- ELISA (HSV, VZV, CMV) Aqueous or vitreous fluid
- Polymerase chain reaction (PCR) HSV, VZV, CMV

Treatment

- Antiviral therapy—Intravenous acyclovir initially followed by oral acyclovir.
- Prophylactic laser photocoagulation may help prevent retinal detachment.

REFERENCES

1. Yoser SL, Forster DJ, Rao NA. Systemic viral infections and their retinal and choroidal manifestation. Surv Ophthalmol. 1993; 37: 313-352.
2. Biswas J, Madhavan HN, Gopal L, Badrinath SS: Clinical features and virologic studies in viral retinitis. Ind J Ophthalmol 1995;43: 63-68.
3. Ganatra JB, Chandler D, Santos C, *et al*. Viral causes of the acute retinal necrosis syndrome. Am J Ophthalmol 2000; 129:166–172.

Acute Retinal Necrosis

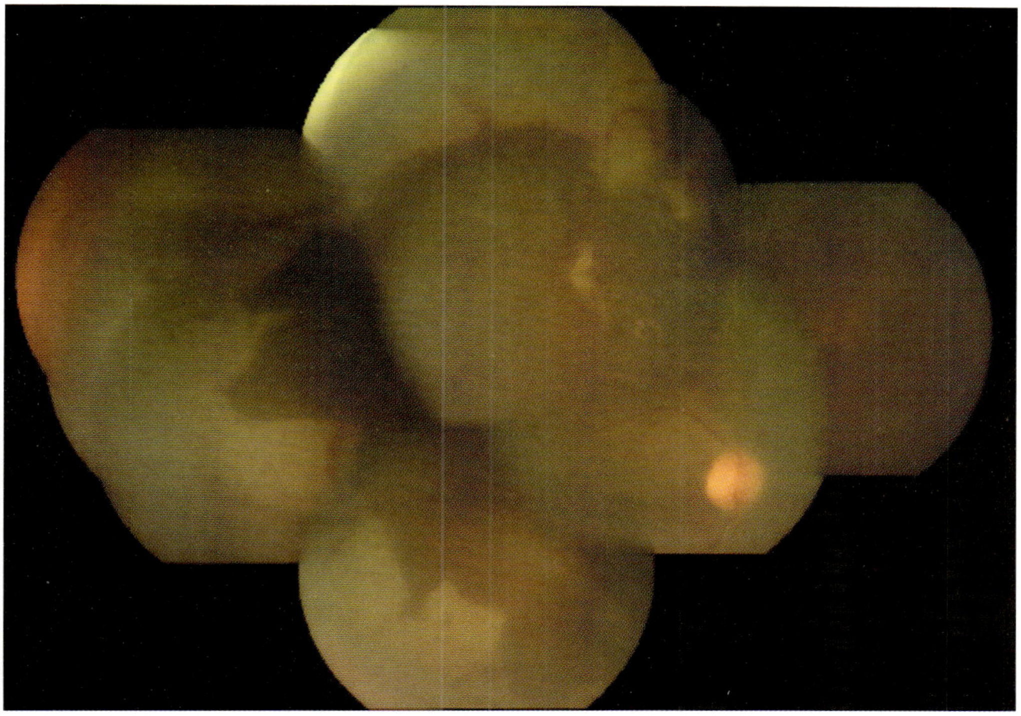

Fig. 16.1: Fundus photograph of a patient with acute retinal necrosis showing vitritis, vasculitis and yellowish white retinitis with scalloped margins in the peripheral retina

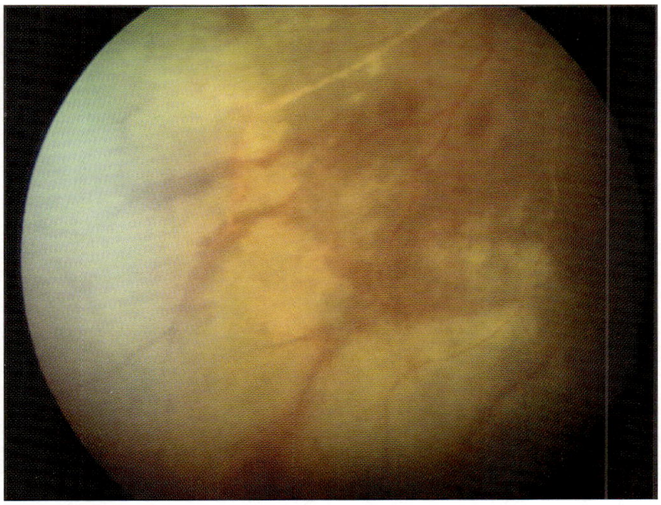

Fig. 16.2: Necrosis of peripheral retina with sheathing of vessels in acute retinal necrosis

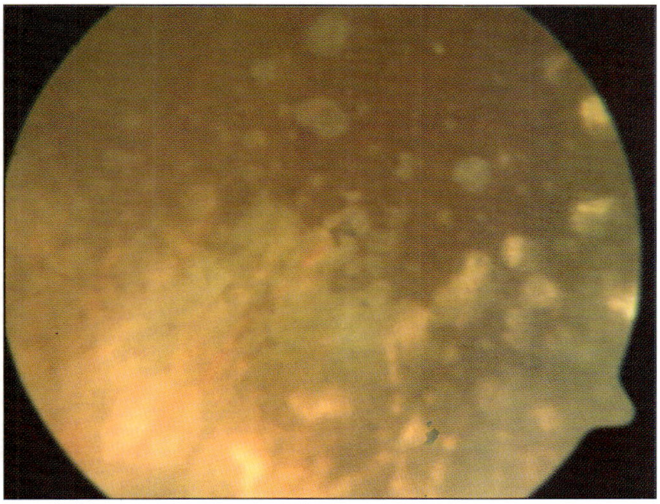

Fig. 16.3: Regression of retinal necrosis showing classical 'swiss cheeselike pattern' following intravenous acyclovir therapy

A 25-year-old patient presented to our clinic with complaints of pain, redness and decreased vision in the left eye for 2 days. His vision was counting fingers at 2 m. Slit lamp evaluation showed aqueous cells and flare as well as vitreous cells.

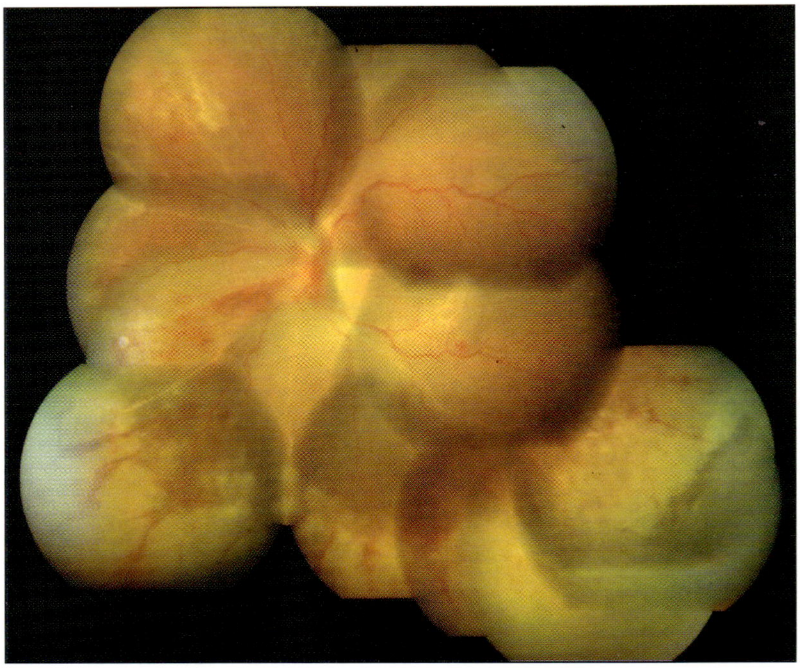

Fig. 16.4: Fundus examination revealed disc edema, vasculitis, retinal hemorrhages and areas of retinal necrosis in the periphery. Inferotemporal quadrant showed large retinal break. Anterior chamber tap was done and multiplex polymerase chain reaction for varicella zoster virus was positive in the aqueous aspirate

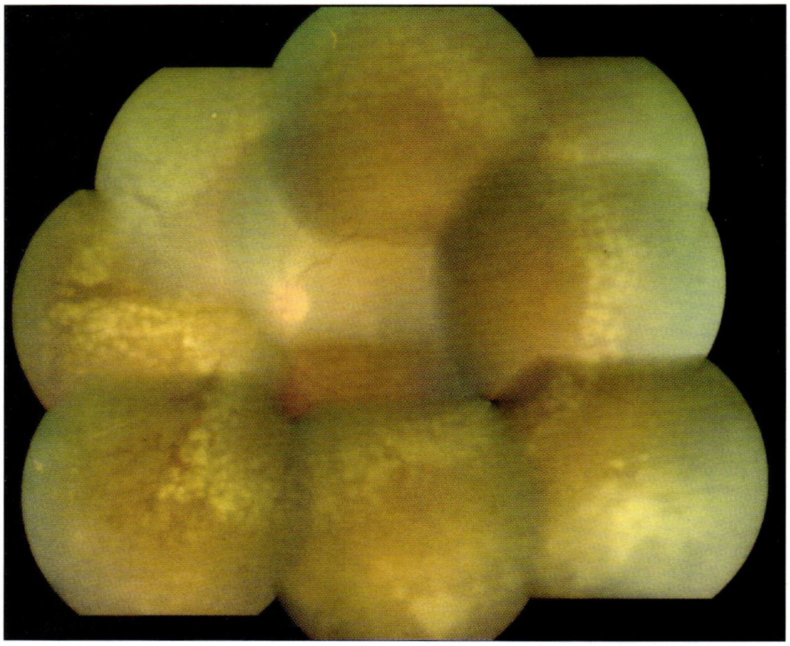

Fig. 16.5: Montage fundus photograph following treatment with intravenous acyclovir and barrage laser photocoagulation

Complications of ARN

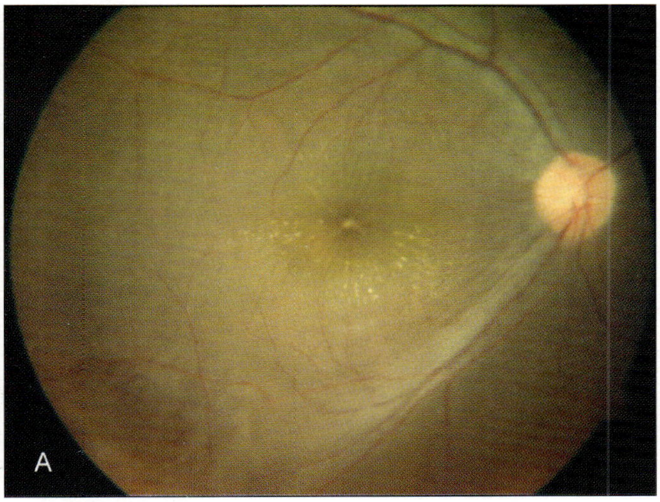

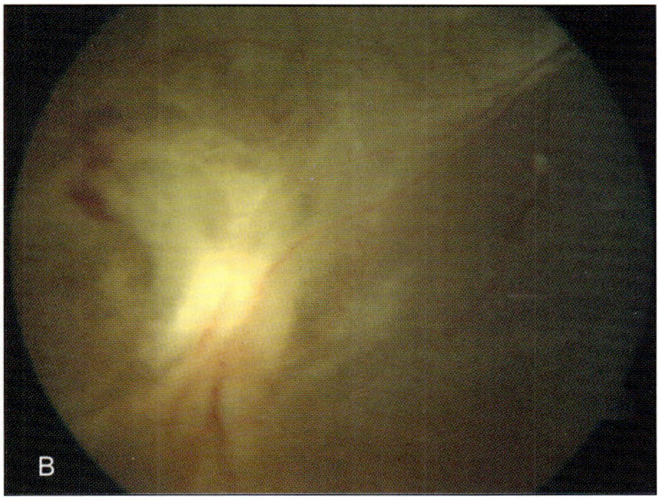

Figs 16.6A and B: Combined rhegmatogenous and tractional retinal detachment in a patient with acute retinal necrosis

Necrotizing Herpetic Retinopathy (HSV or VZV)

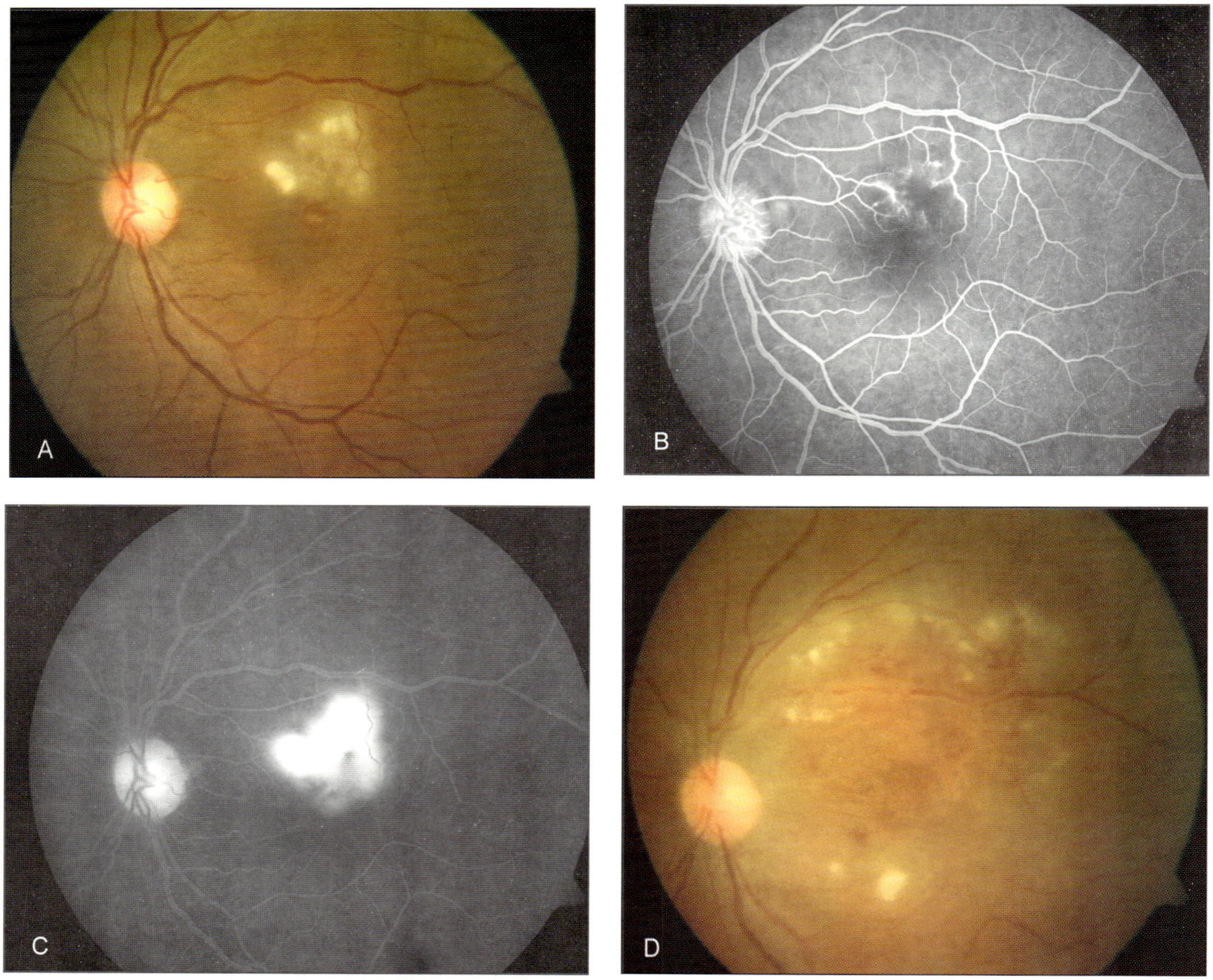

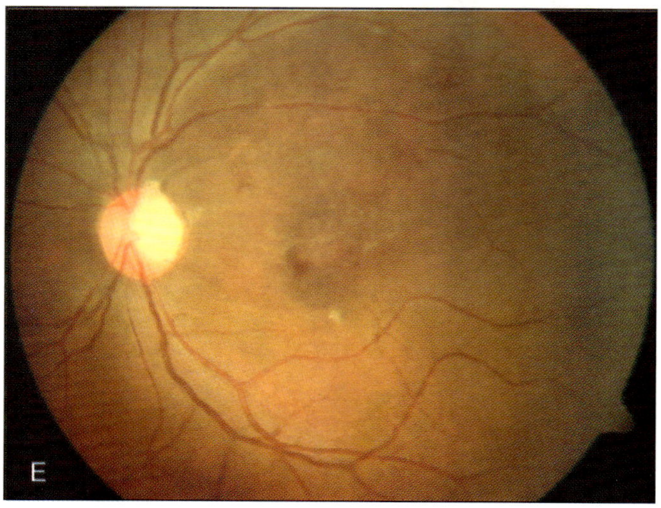

Figs 16.7A to E: A 35-year-old lady came with complaints of sudden decrease in vision in left eye since 1 week. (A) Fundus examination showed yellowish white retinal infiltrates with cuffs of vasculitis close to fovea. (B and C) Fluorescein angiogram revealed arteriolar occlusion, vascular staining and areas of capillary nonperfusion with leakage of the dye in the late phase. (D and E) Viral serology was positive for *varicella zoster virus* and subsequently intravenous acyclovir was started following which complete resolution of the lesions was noted

A 17-year-old male complained of sudden diminution of vision in both eyes since 10 days. Visual acuity in both eyes was counting fingers one meter

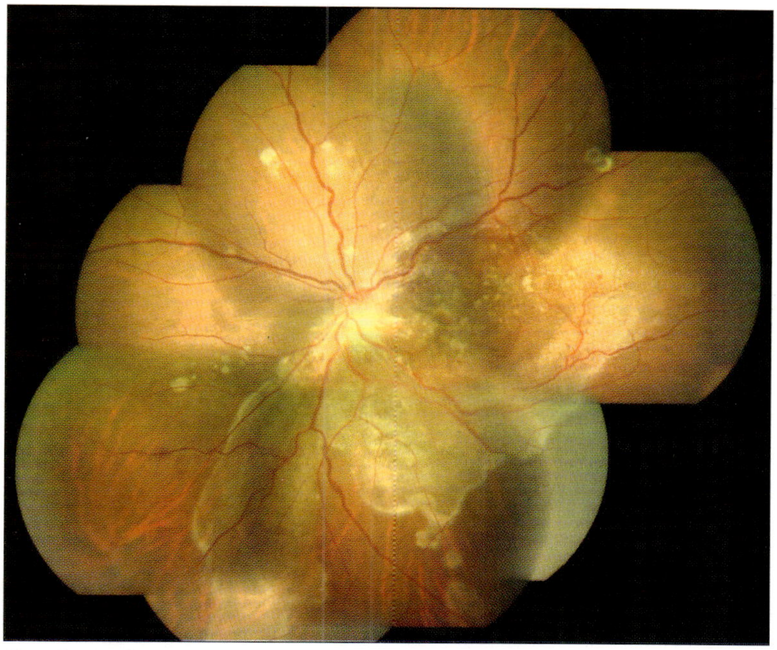

Fig. 16.8: Fundus examination revealed extensive outer retinal necrosis involving the macula with sparing of the retinal vessels. Viral serology showed raised titers of IgG for HSV and VZV. Patient was treated with intravenous acyclovir and oral acyclovir

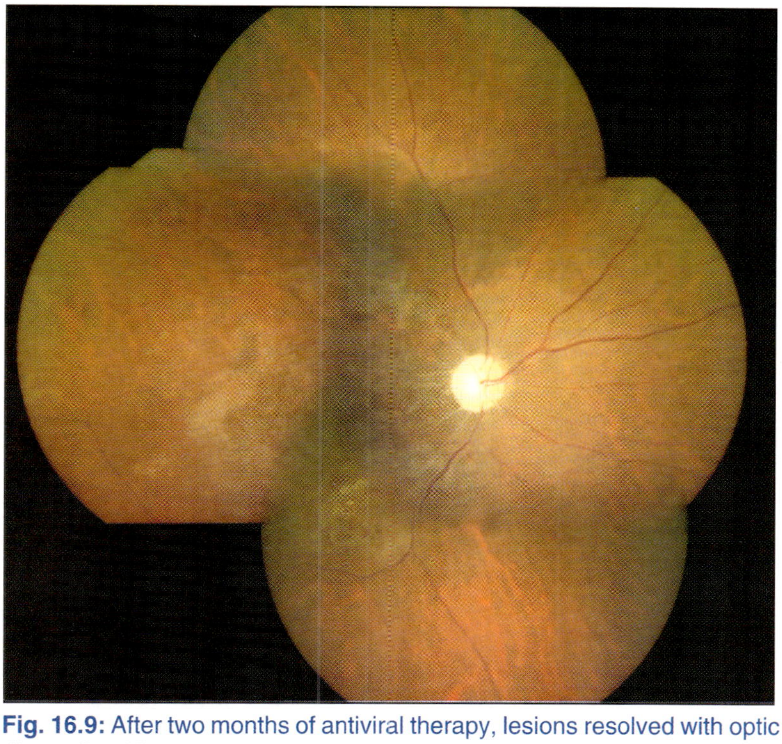

Fig. 16.9: After two months of antiviral therapy, lesions resolved with optic disc pallor. Visual acuity in both eyes was 6/60

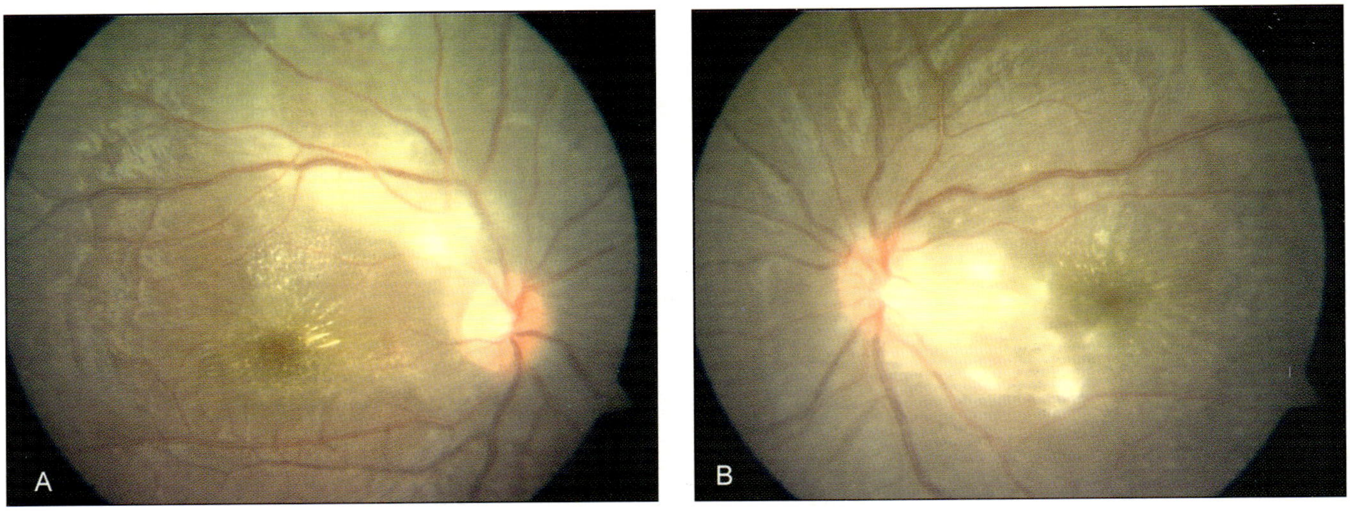

Figs 16.10A and B: Fundus photograph of right and left eye of a 12-year-old boy showing areas of necrotizing viral retinitis with neuroretinitis

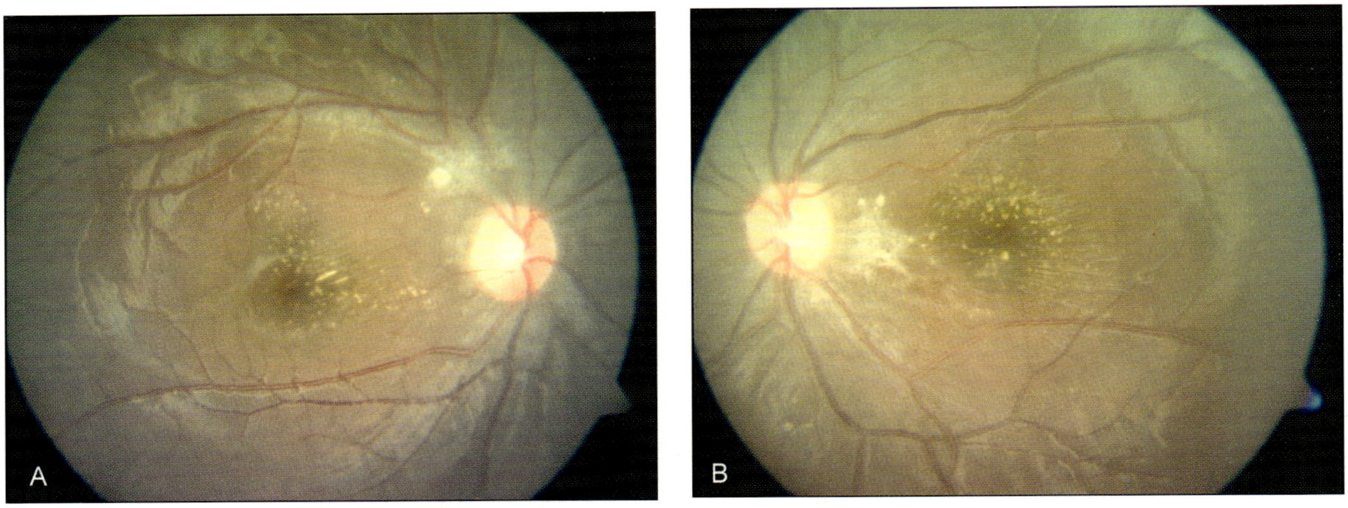

Figs 16.11A and B: Resolved viral retinitis following treatment with oral acyclovir therapy

CHAPTER SEVENTEEN

Retinal Vasculitis

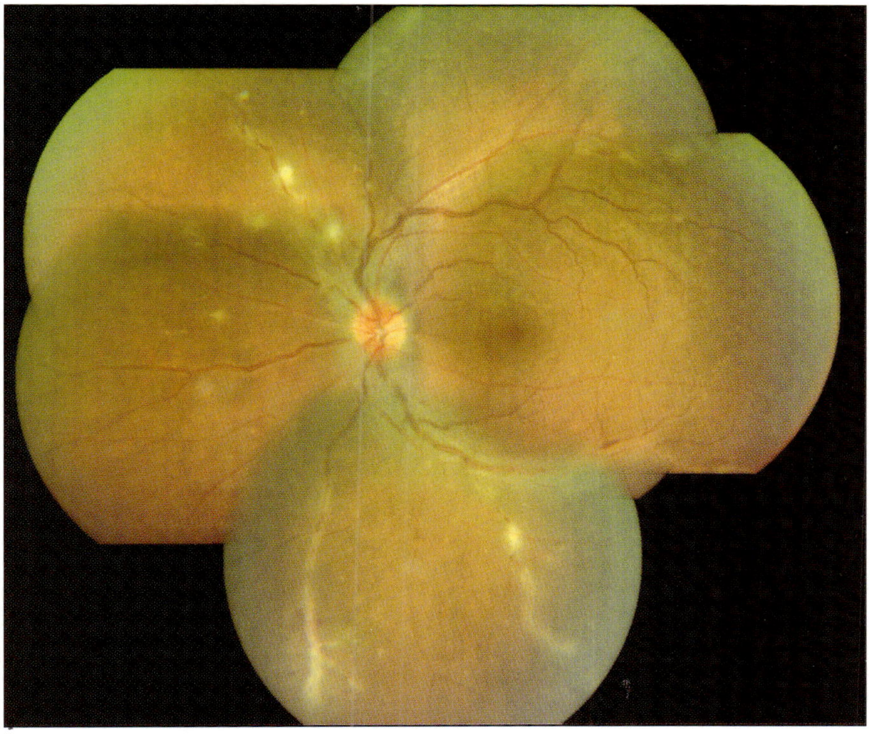

Retinal vasculitis is defined as inflammation of the retinal vessels associated with intraocular inflammation. The term 'vasculitis' is a misnomer. This clinically noted pathologic condition is better termed perivasculitis or phlebitis due to the exudative gray white sheathing of the blood vessels mainly retinal veins. Retinal vasculitis usually occurs in association with ocular or systemic diseases. It usually affects young adults between 15-40 years of age.

Various ocular diseases presenting with retinal vasculitis are:

1. *Non-infective*
   - Ocular diseasess, Idiopathic, Eales disease, intermediate uveitis, frosted branch angiitis
   - *Systemic diseases:* Behcet's disease, sarcoidosis, SLE, Wegener's granulomatosis, malignancy
2. *Infective:* Toxoplasmosis, tuberculosis, syphilis, herpes simplex, herpes zoster, cytomegalovirus, AIDS

Ocular Features

Symptoms

Blurred vision, floaters, scotoma.

Signs

- Anterior uveitis
- Vitreitis
- Focal areas of fluffy white sheathing as well as skip lesions
- Exaggerated areas of sheathing as **frosted branch angiitis**
- Retinal hemorrhages, cystoid macular edema, optic disc edema
- Vitreous hemorrhage

Complications

Branch vein occlusion, macular ischemia, retinal or disc neovascularization, tractional retinal detachment.

Systemic Features

Oral or genital ulcers, arthritis, skin ulcerations, neurologic or respiratory disease.

Investigations

FFA

- Vascular staining and leakage, capillary nonperfusion, retinal neovascularization, cystoid macular edema, optic disc leak
- Nerve fiber layer infarcts

Laboratory investigations

- Complete blood count
- Erythrocyte sedimentation rate
- C-reactive protein
- Basic coagulation profile
- VDRL/TPHA
- Mantoux test
- Serum angiotensin converting enzyme
- Collagen work up—Rheumatoid factor, antinuclear antibody, antineutrophillic cytoplasmic antibody.
- Antiphospholipid antibodies
- Chest X-ray

Treatment

1. Corticosteroids—Periocular, systemic.
2. Immunosuppressives—Azathioprine, Cyclosporine, Mycophenolate mofetil.
3. Laser photocoagulation—In cases of retinal neovascularization and significant capillary closure.
4. Vitrectomy—Nonclearing vitreous hemorrhage, tractional retinal detachment.

REFERENCES

1. Foster CS, Regan CDJ. Retinal vascular disease: Management. IOC Summer 1991;31:3:55-71.
2. George RK, Walton RC, Whitcup SM, Nussenblatt RB. Primary retinal vasculitis: Systemic associations and diagnostic evaluation. Ophthalmology 1996;103:384-389.
3. Walton C, Ashmore E. Retinal vasculitis. Curr Opin Ophthalmol 2003;14:413-419.
4. Narayana KM, Agrawal R, Biswas J, Arjundas D. Recurrent anterior uveitis and healed retinal vasculitis associated with multiple sclerosis. Ind J Ophthalmol 2003;51:77-79.

Idiopathic Retinal Vasculitis

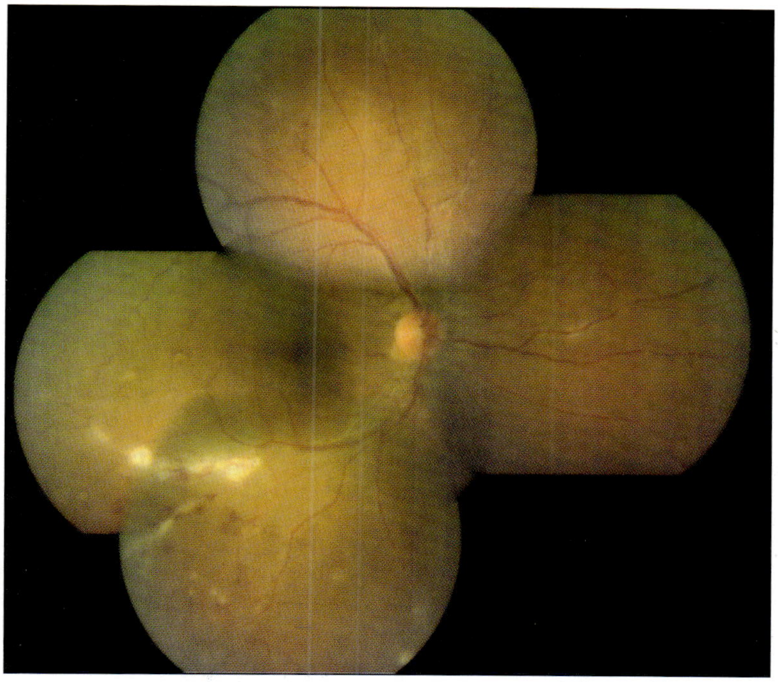

Fig. 17.1: Fundus photograph of a patient with acute retinal vasculitis showing multiple areas of perivascular cuffing with few retinal hemorrages along the inferior temporal arcade.The collection of inflammatory cells within and around the vessels gives the appearance of cuffing

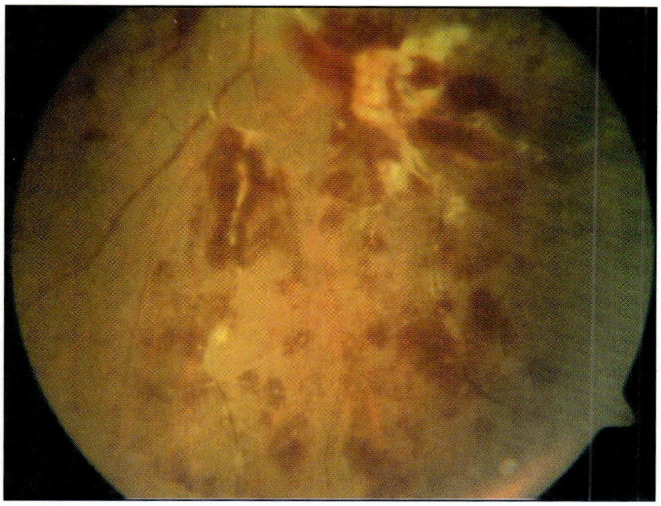

Fig. 17.2: Extensive periphlebitis with exudation and retinal hemorrhages involving the inferior peripheral retina (Branch retinal vein occlusion following inflammation)

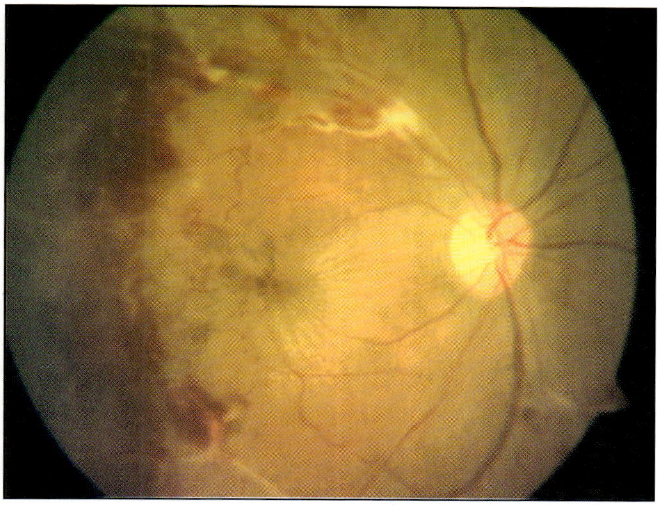

Fig. 17.3: Retinal vasculitis involving the posterior pole with star exudates in the macula (Central Eales' disease)

Complications of Vasculitis

Capillary nonperfusion

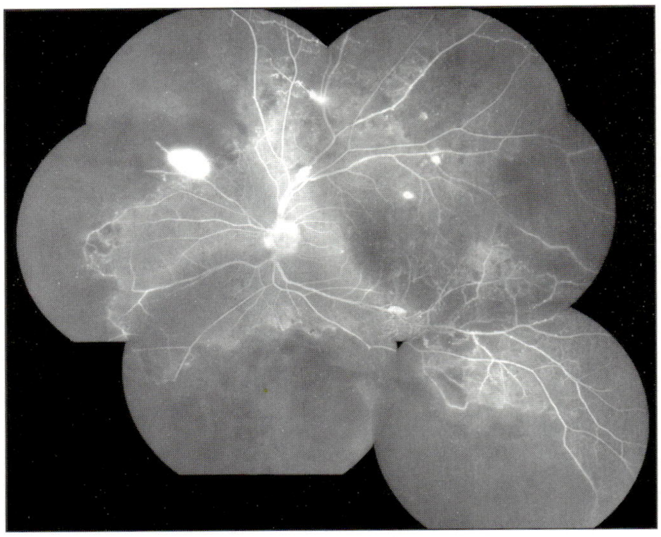

Fig. 17.4: Montage of fluorescein angiogram of a patient with Eales' disease showing extensive areas of capillary nonperfusion in the periphery

Retinal neovascularization elsewhere

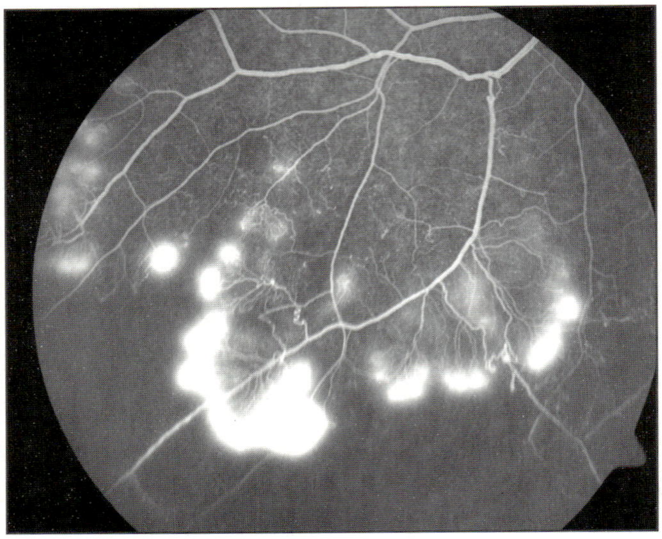

Fig. 17.5: Late phase angiogram of the same patient showing profuse leakage due to retinal neovascularization.

Neovascularization of the disc

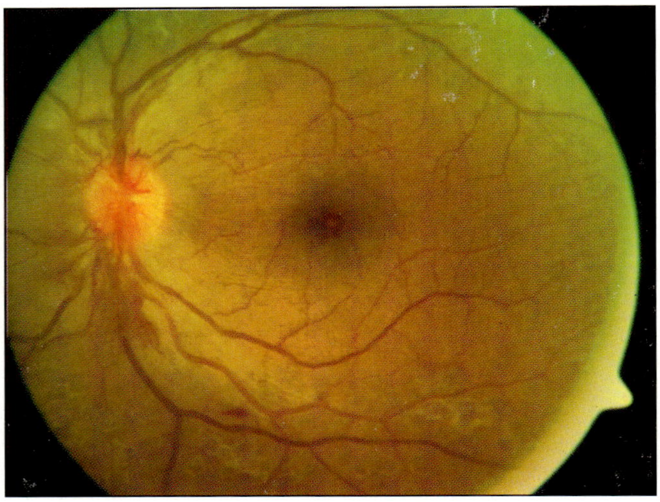

Fig. 17.6: Disc neovascularization and cystoid macular edema in a patient with Eales' disease

Cystoid macular edema

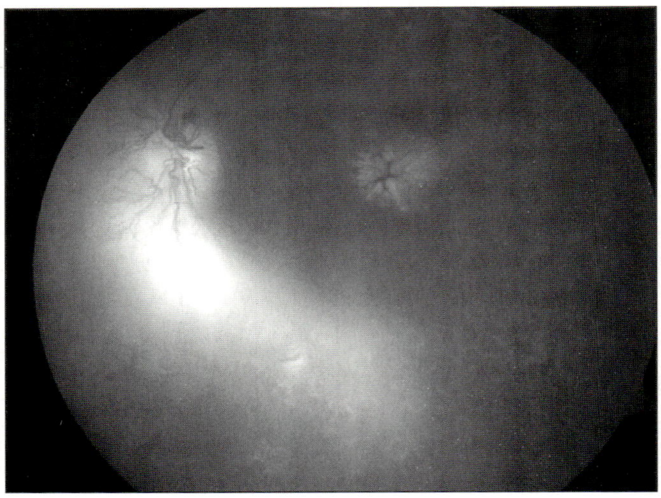

Fig. 17.7: Fluorescein angiogram of the same patient showing disc leakage and petalloid hyperfluorescence suggestive of cystoid macular edema

Vasculitis associated with Infections

Vasculitis in CMV retinitis

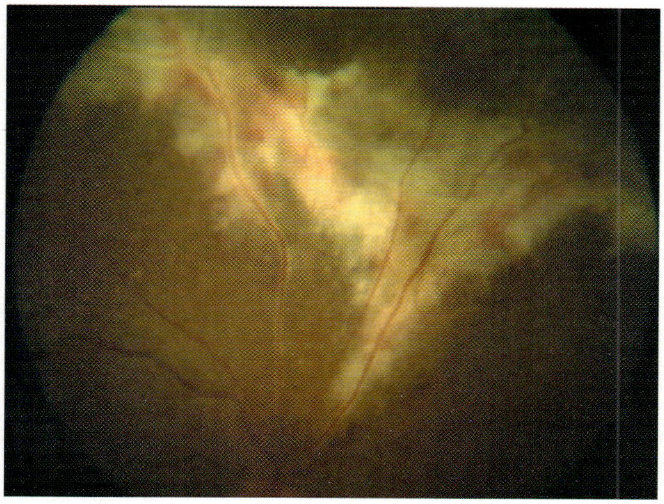

Fig. 17.8: Fundus photograph of a patient with CMV retinitis showing dense white fluffy retinal infitrates, retinal hemorrhages and perivasculitis

Vasculitis in toxoplasmic retinochoroiditis

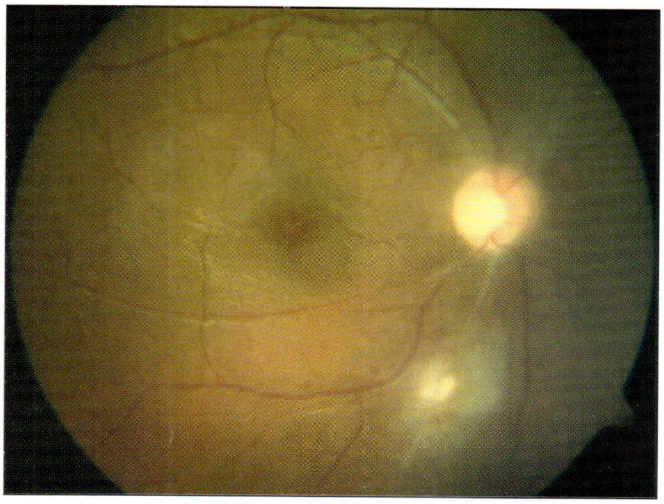

Fig. 17.9: Fundus of a patient with toxoplasmic retinochoroiditis showing active vasculitis surrounding the lesion

Vasculitis in herpetic retinitis

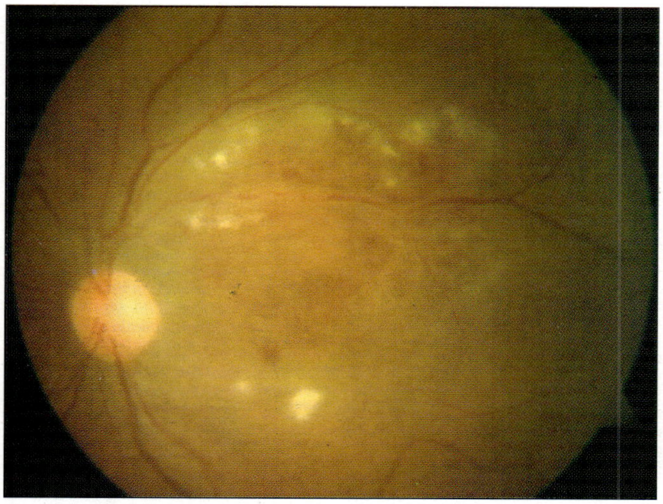

Fig. 17.10: Fundus photograph showing yellowish white retinal necrotic lesions with periarteritis causing macular branch arteriolar occlusion

Vasculitis in tuberculosis

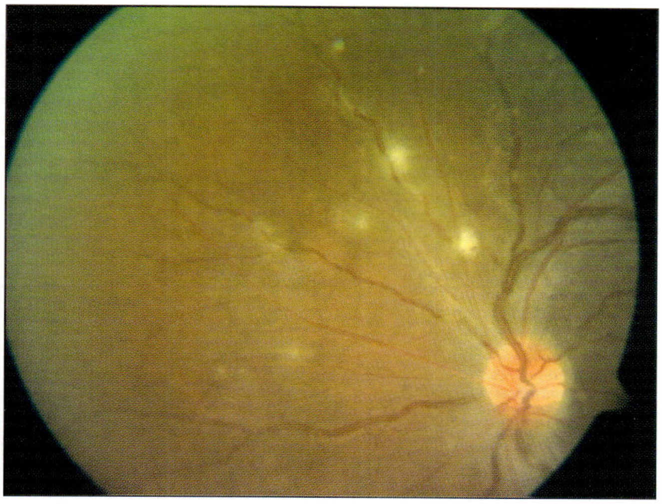

Fig. 17.11: Retinal periphlebitis with multiple areas of vascular cuffing in a patient with pulmonary tuberculosis

Idiopathic Frosted Branch Angiitis

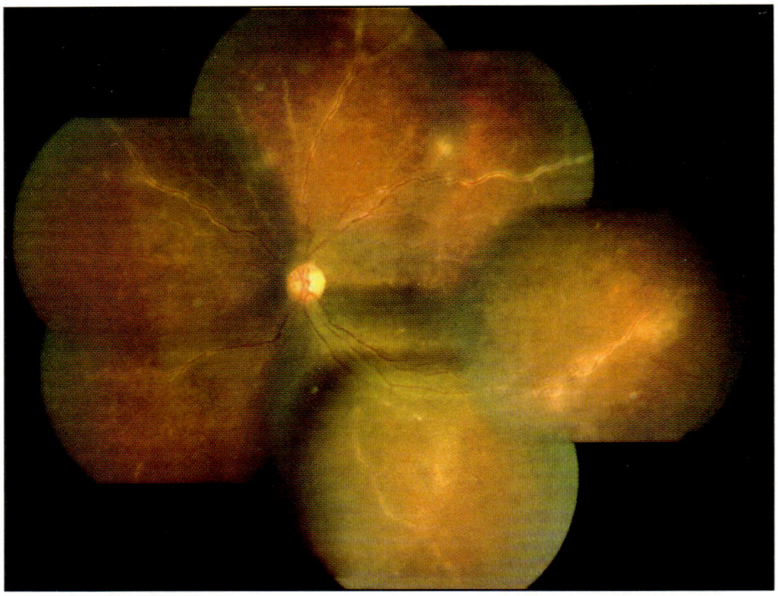

Fig. 17.12: Frosted branch angiitis in a 30-year-old immunocompetent patient. Vasculitis resolved completely with a course of oral steroids

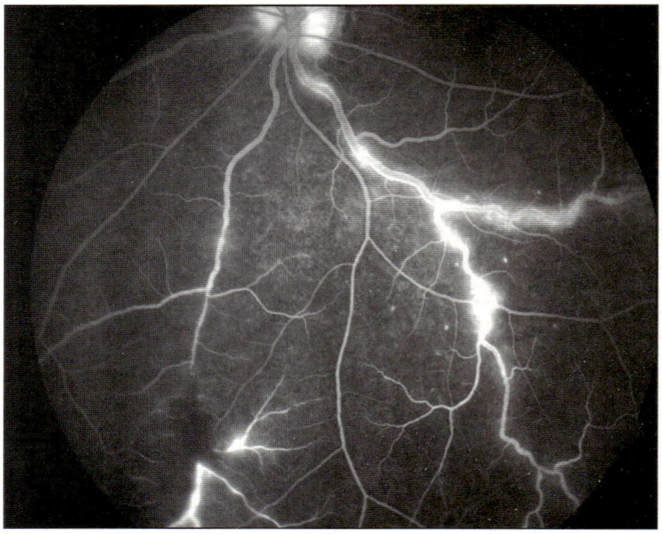

Fig. 17.13: Late phase fluorescein angiogram demonstrating staining of blood vessel walls in retinal vasculitis

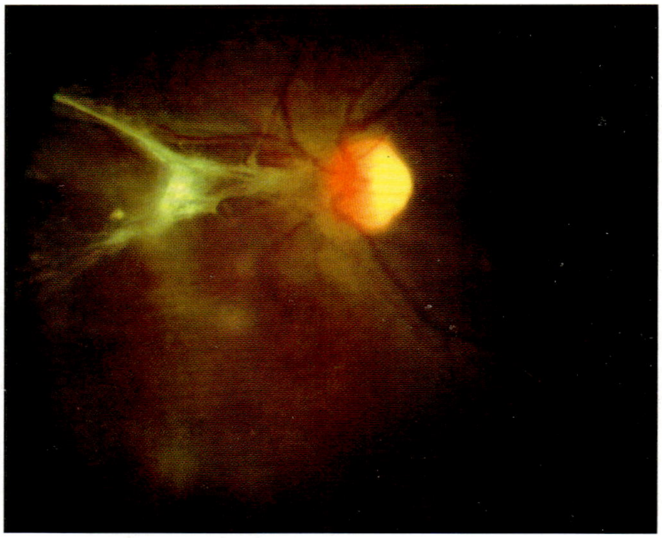

Fig. 17.14: Proliferative vitreoretinopathy following chronic vasculitis and vitreous inflammation

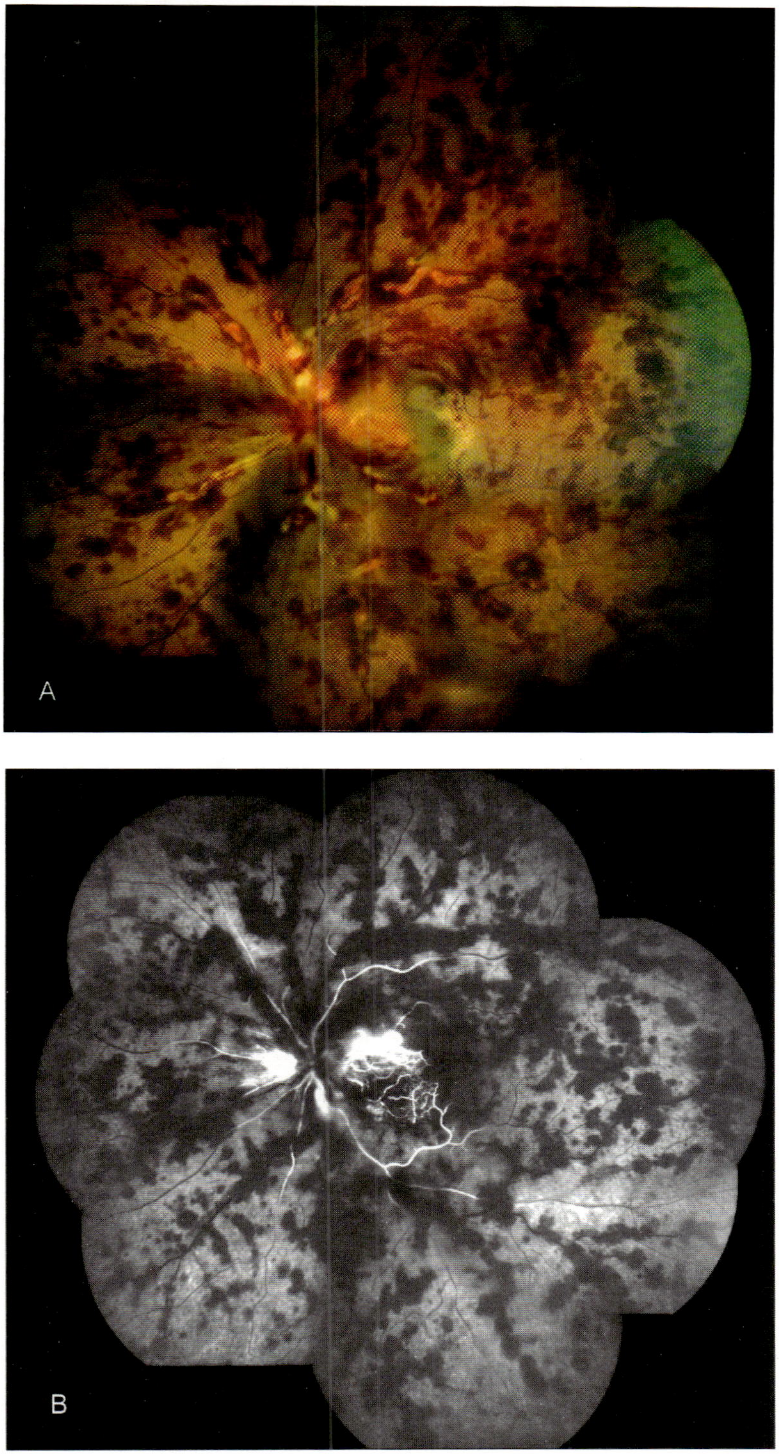

Figs 17.15A and B: Central retinal vein occlusion leading to hemorrhagic retinopathy in a patient with sarcoidosis

Section 4
Panuveitis

CHAPTER EIGHTEEN

Sarcoidosis

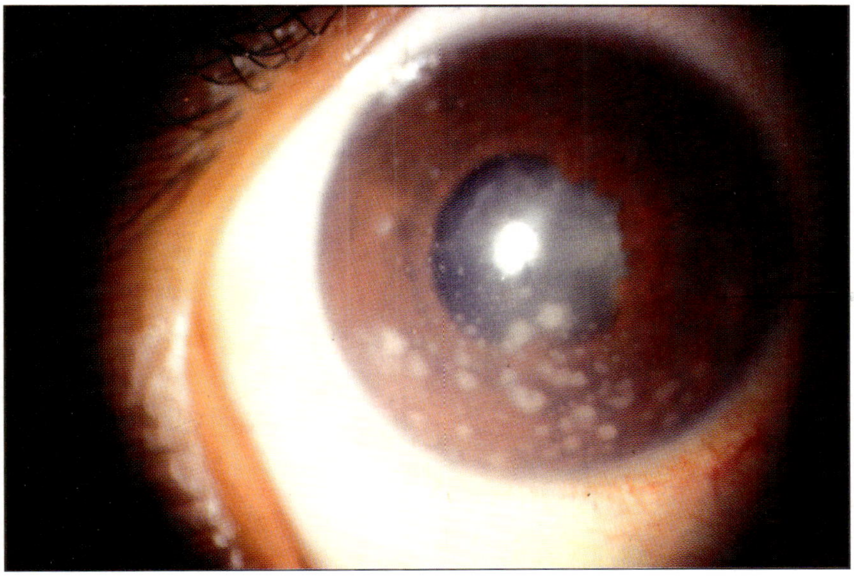

Sarcoidosis is a chronic multisystem granulomatous disease of unknown etiology. It occurs worldwide but is more common in US blacks, Scandinavian and Irish white population. It primarily affects adults in the age group 20-50 years but may also be seen in children and elderly. Sarcoidosis affects lungs, thoracic lymph nodes, skin and eyes. Ocular involvement is seen in 25-60 percent of patients with systemic sarcoidosis.

Ocular Features

- Lacrimal gland: Keratoconjunctiva sicca
- Conjunctival nodules
- Uveitis:
  - Anterior: Granulomatous, mutton fat keratic precipitates, Koeppe and Bussaca nodules, cataract, glaucoma.
  - Intermediate: Snowball exudates and snow banking in pars plana
  - Posterior: Vitritis, periphlebitis, candle wax drippings (Taches de bougies), choroidal granulomas

    Disc granuloma, retrobulbar optic neuritis, optic atrophy

    Hemorrhagic retinopathy, arterial macro-aneurysms

Complications

Cystoid macular edema, cataract, glaucoma, retinal ischemia, neovascularization

Systemic Features

Lungs

Stage I: Bilateral hilar lymphadenopathy.

Stage II: Bilateral hilar lymphadenopathy with parenchymal involvement.

Stage III: Lung infiltration only.

Stage IV: Lung fibrosis.

Skin: Nodules, plaques, psoriasiform lesions, ulcerations, lupus pernio, erythema nodosum

Joints: Arthritis.

Heart: Arrhythmias, conduction defects.

Investigations

- Serum ACE and lysozyme
- Serum calcium, phosphorus
- Mantoux test
- Chest X-ray
- CT scan chest
- Whole body Gallium scans
- Bronchoalveolar lavage
- Biopsy—Histopathology shows non-caseating granulomas with large central nodules of epithelioid cells surrounded by lymphocytes and mononuclear cells.

Treatment

Corticosteroids and immunosuppressives (methotrexate, azathioprine, cyclosporine).

REFERENCES

1. De Rosa AJ, Margo CE, Orlick ME. Hemorrhagic retinopathy as a presenting manifestation of sarcoidosis. Retina 1995;15:422- 427.
2. Dev S, McCallum RM, Jaffe GJ. Methotrexate treatment for sarcoid associated panuveitis. Ophthalmology 1999; 106:111-18.
3. Rothova A. Ocular involvement in sarcoidosis. Br J Ophthalmol 2000;84;110-16.
4. Uyama M. Uveitis in sarcoidosis. Int Ophthalmol Clin 2002; 42:143-50.

Ocular Manifestations of Sarcoidosis

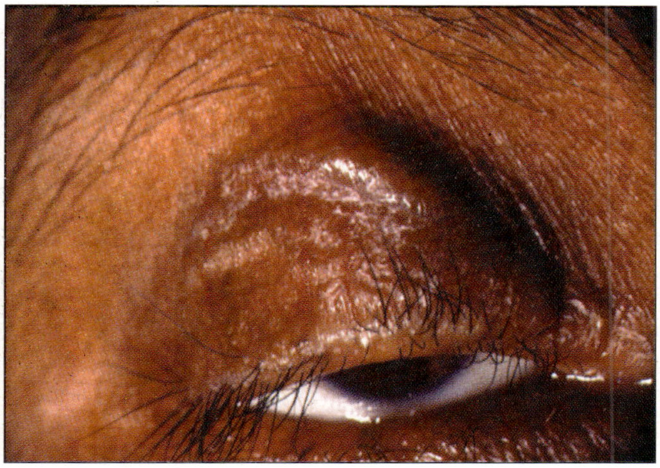

Fig. 18.1: Sarcoid granuloma involving the upper lid

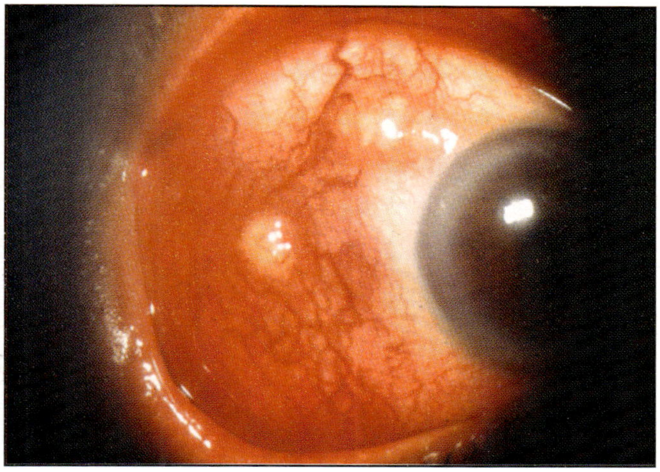

Fig. 18.2: Conjunctival nodules in sarcoidosis, biopsy of which showed noncaseating granuloma

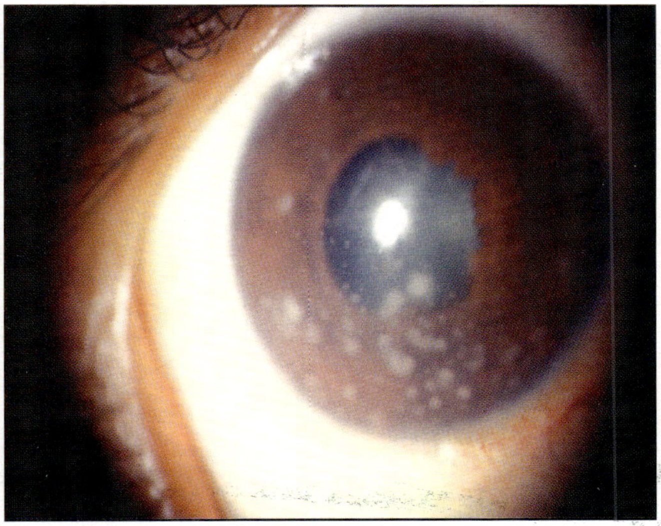

Fig. 18.3: Sarcoid anterior uveitis showing white mutton fat keratic precipitates, iris nodules, posterior synechiae and complicated cataract

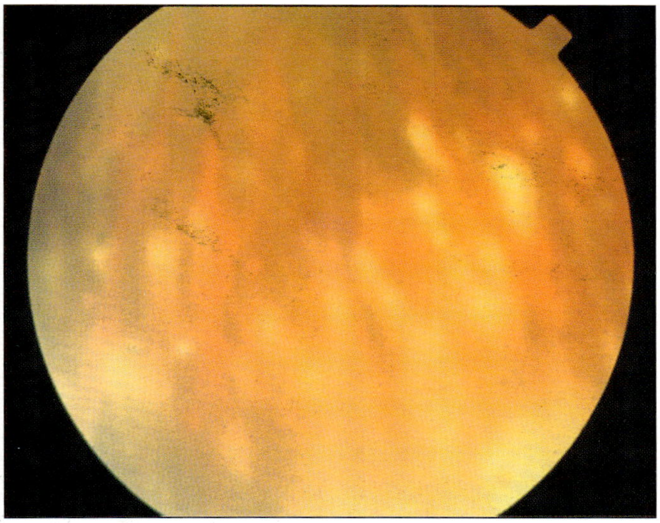

Fig. 18.4: Snowballs in the vitreous cavity in a patient with sarcoidosis

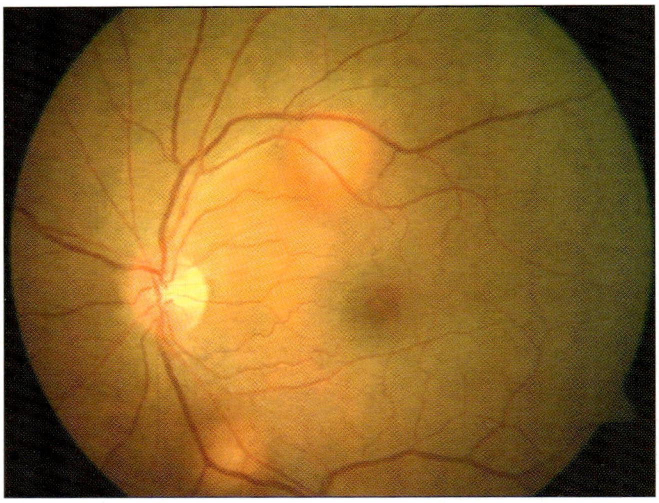

Fig. 18.5: Yellowish round subretinal nodules presenting as choroidal granulomas in sarcoidosis

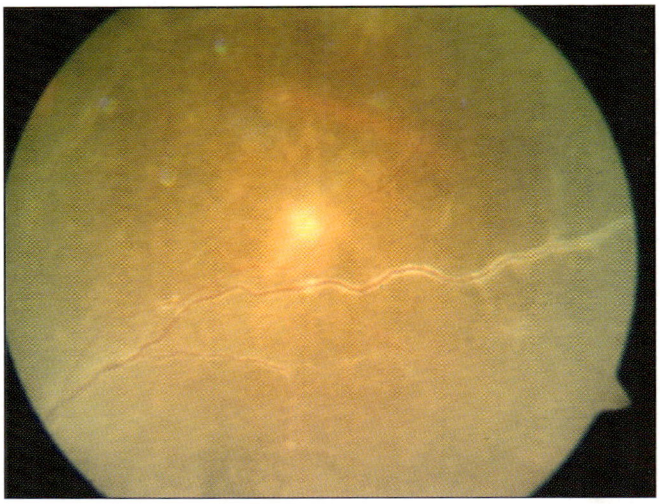

Fig. 18.6: Candle wax like exudation around a peripheral retinal vein

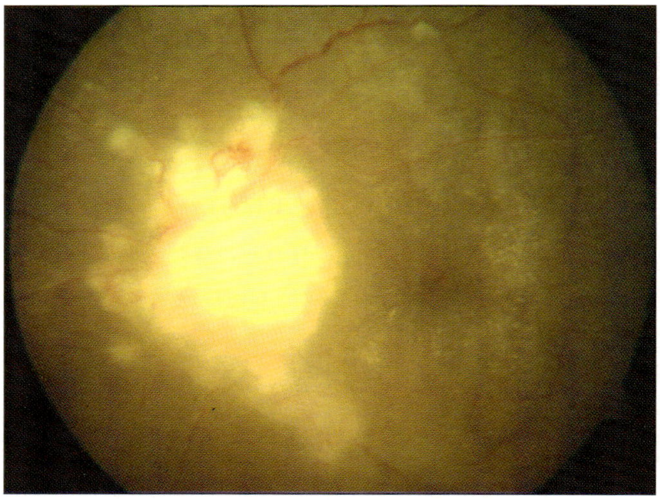

Fig. 18.7: Optic nerve head granuloma with neuroretinitis in a patient with sarcoidosis

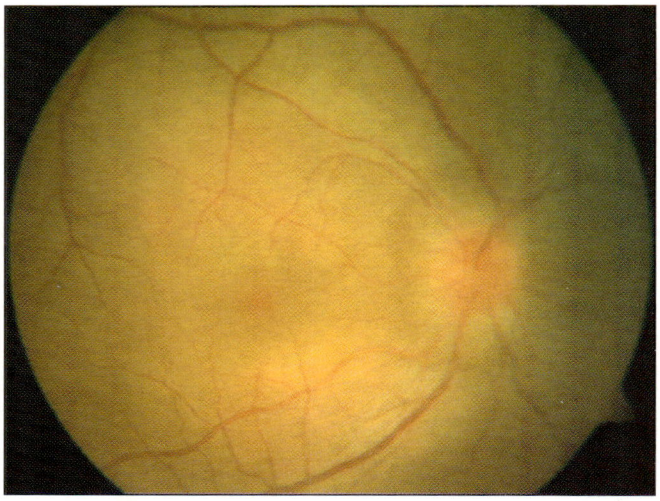

Fig. 18.8: Fundus photograph of a patient with sarcoidosis showing disc edema. Pars plana showed snowball exudates in the inferior quadrant

Systemic Manifestatons of Sarcoidosis

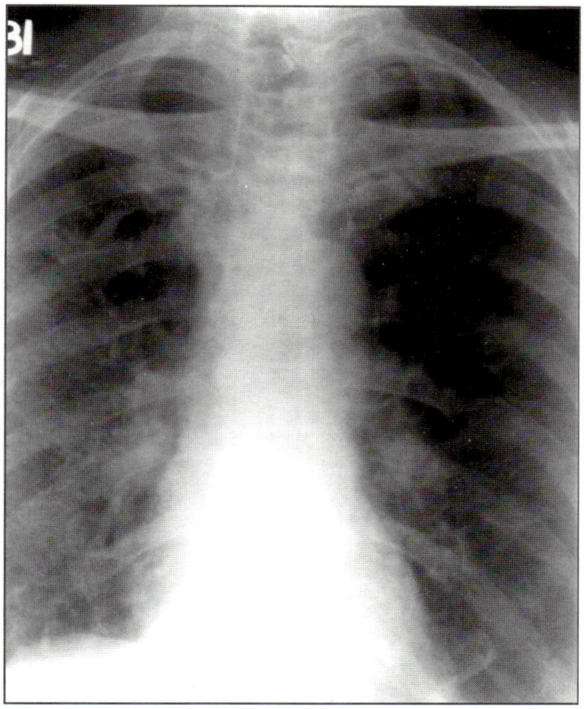

Fig. 18.9: Chest X-ray showing bilateral hilar lymphadenopathy in a patient with sarcoid uveitis

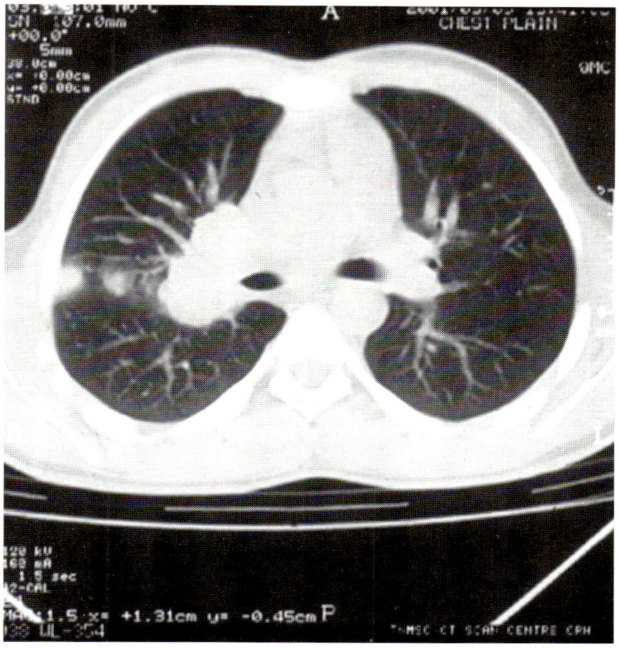

Fig. 18.10: CT chest in a patient with sarcoidosis showing enlarged hilar shadows

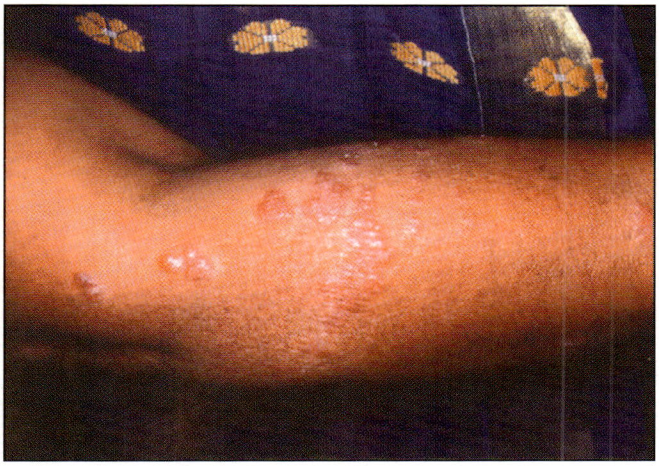

Fig. 18.11: Erythematous plaque like lesions on the forearm in a patient with ocular sarcoidosis

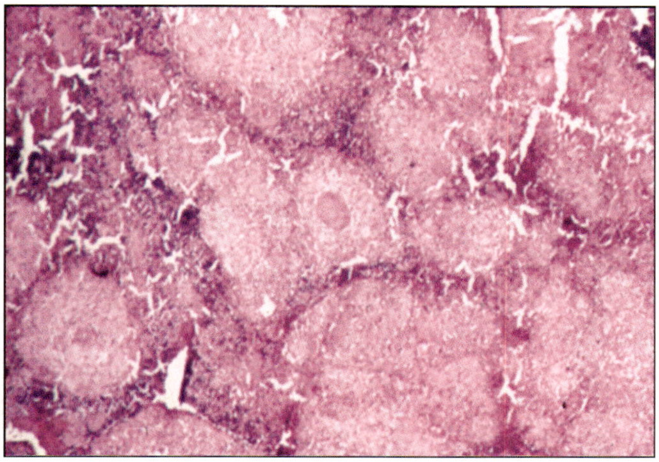

Fig. 18.12: Histopathology of the skin lesions showed multiple noncaseating granulomas

CHAPTER NINETEEN

Vogt-Koyanagi-Harada (VKH) Syndrome

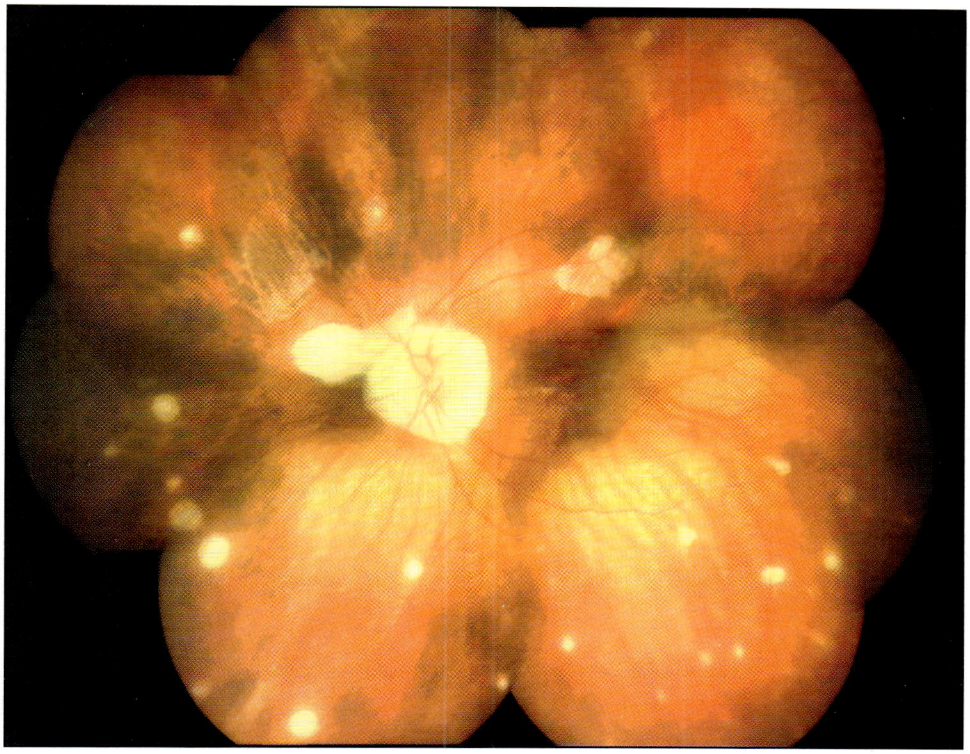

VKH is a severe bilateral granulomatous panuveitis which also affects skin, hair, inner ear and meninges. It is a T-cell mediated autoimmune process directed against melanin containing cells of uvea, meninges, inner ear and dermal melanocytes. It occurs more commonly in East and Southeast Asians, Asian Indians, Middle Easterners, Native Americans and Hispanics. It is seen usually in third and fifth decades.

Clinical Features

1. Prodromal phase: Headache, fever, malaise, nausea, nuchal rigidity, tinnitus, dysacousia, and hearing loss.
2. Acute uveitic phase: Diffuse choroiditis, disc hyperemia and edema, exudative retinal detachment.
3. Chronic phase: Perilimbal vitiligo (Sugiura's sign), sunset glow fundus, rounded chorioretinal depigmented scars (Dalen-Fuchs nodules).
   Alopecia, poliosis, vitiligo
4. Chronic recurrent phase iridocyclitis and complications like cataract, glaucoma, choroidal neovascular membrane, subretinal fibrosis.

Investigations

FFA

- Multiple areas of pinpoint leaks in the early phase followed by large placoid areas of hyperfluorescence and pooling of dye within subretinal space.
- Optic nerve head staining.

U/S

- Diffuse choroidal thickening with serous retinal detachment
- Lumbar puncture: CSF pleocytosis

Treatment

- Systemic (oral/intravenous) and topical corticosteroids
- Immunosuppressives

REFERENCES

1. Moorthy RS, Inomata H, Rao NA. Vogt Koyanagi Harada syndrome. Surv Ophthalmol 1995:39:265-92.
2. Mondkar SV, Biswas J, Ganesh SK. Analysis of 87 cases with Vogt-Koyanagi-Harada Disease. Japanese Journal of Ophthalmology 2000;44:296-301.
3. Read RW, Holland GN, Rao NA, Tabbara KF, Ohno S, Arellanes-Garcia L, et al. Revised diagnostic criteria for Vogt Koyanagi Harada disease: report of an International Committee on Nomenclature. Am J Ophthalmol 2001;131:647-52.
4. Read RW. Vogt Koyanagi Harada disease. Ophthalmol Clin North Am 2002;15:333-41.
5. Yamaki K, Gocho K, Sakuragi S. Pathogenesis of Vogt-Koyanagi-Harada disease. Int Ophthalmol Clin 2002;42:13-23
6. Ganesh SK, Padmaja MS, Babu K, Biswas J. Cataract surgery in patients with Vogt-Koyanagi-Harada syndrome. J Cataract Refract Surg 2004;30:95-100.

Acute VKH

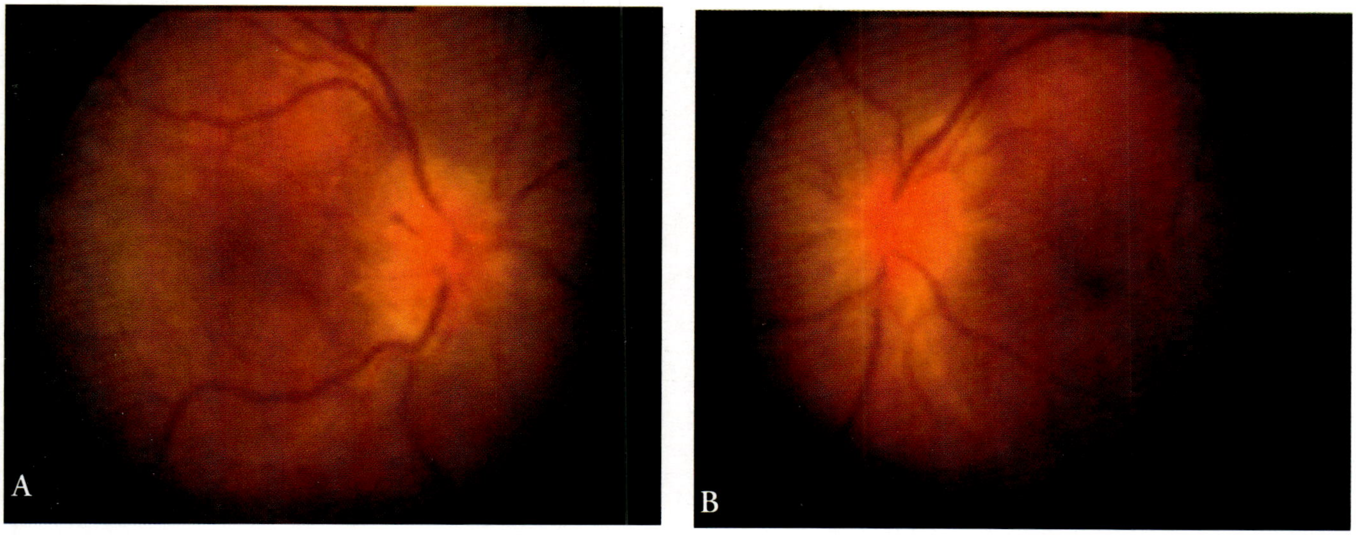

Figs 19.1A and B: Fundus photograph of right and left eye of a patient showing bilateral optic disc edema, hyperemia and exudative retinal detachment in acute uveitic stage of VKH syndrome.

Ultrasound in VKH Syndrome

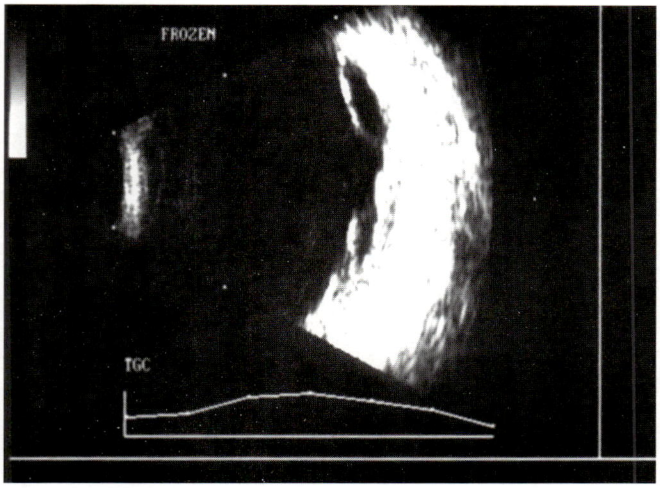

Fig. 19.2: Ultrasound of a patient with VKH syndrome showing serous retinal detachment

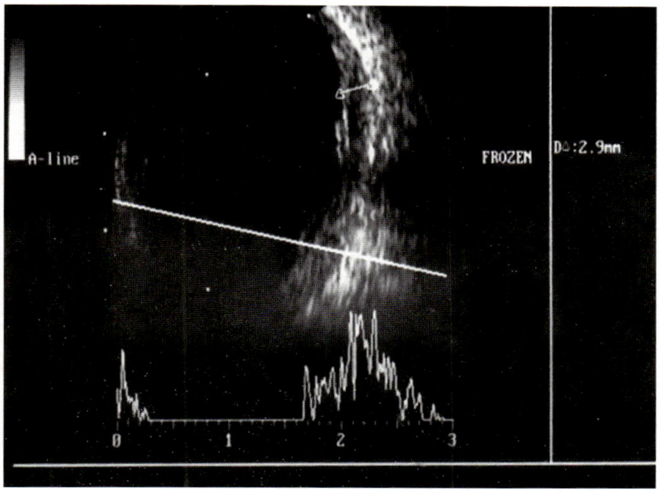

Fig. 19.3: Ultrasound of a patient with VKH syndrome showing diffuse choroidal thickening

Acute VKH

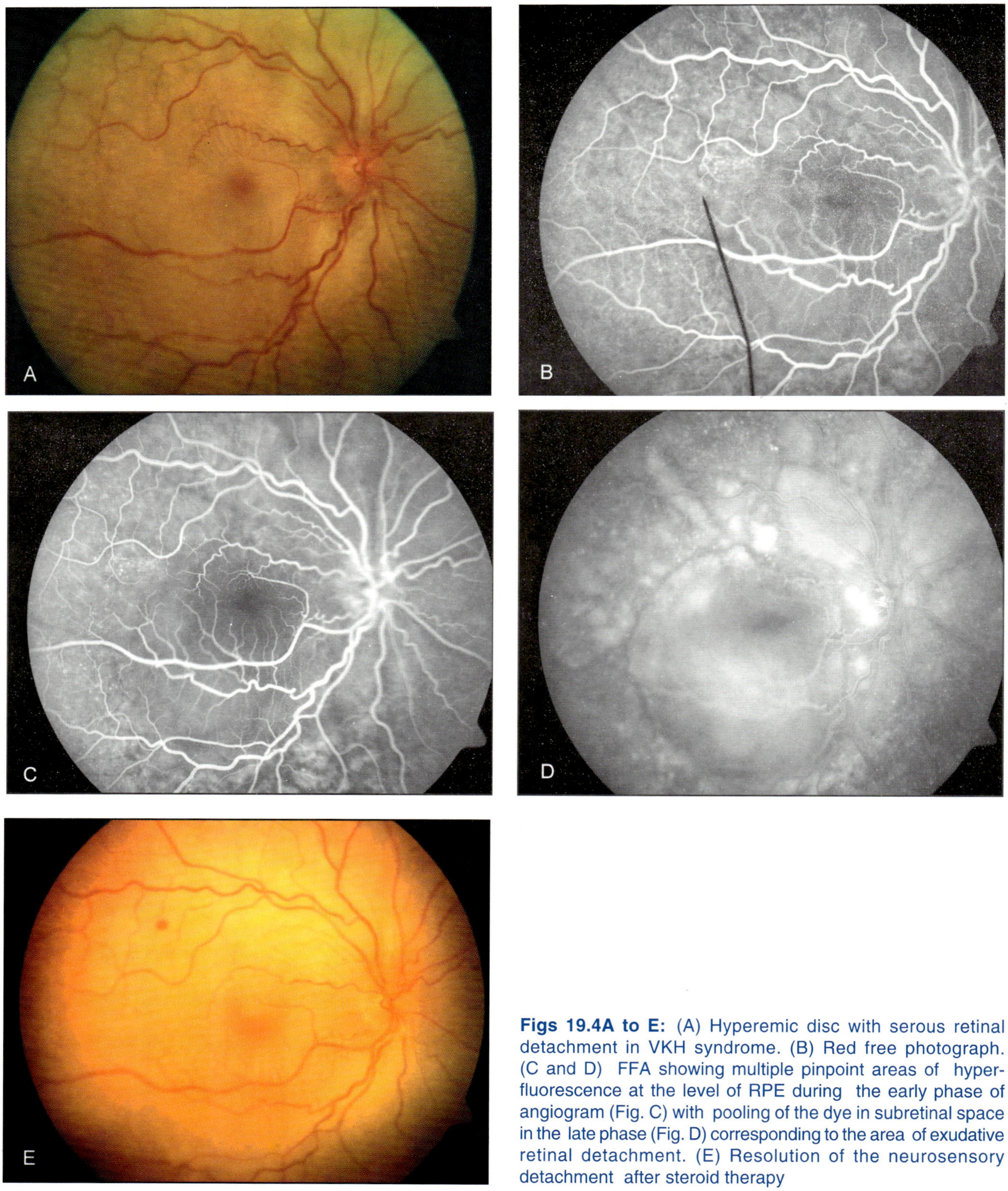

Figs 19.4A to E: (A) Hyperemic disc with serous retinal detachment in VKH syndrome. (B) Red free photograph. (C and D) FFA showing multiple pinpoint areas of hyperfluorescence at the level of RPE during the early phase of angiogram (Fig. C) with pooling of the dye in subretinal space in the late phase (Fig. D) corresponding to the area of exudative retinal detachment. (E) Resolution of the neurosensory detachment after steroid therapy

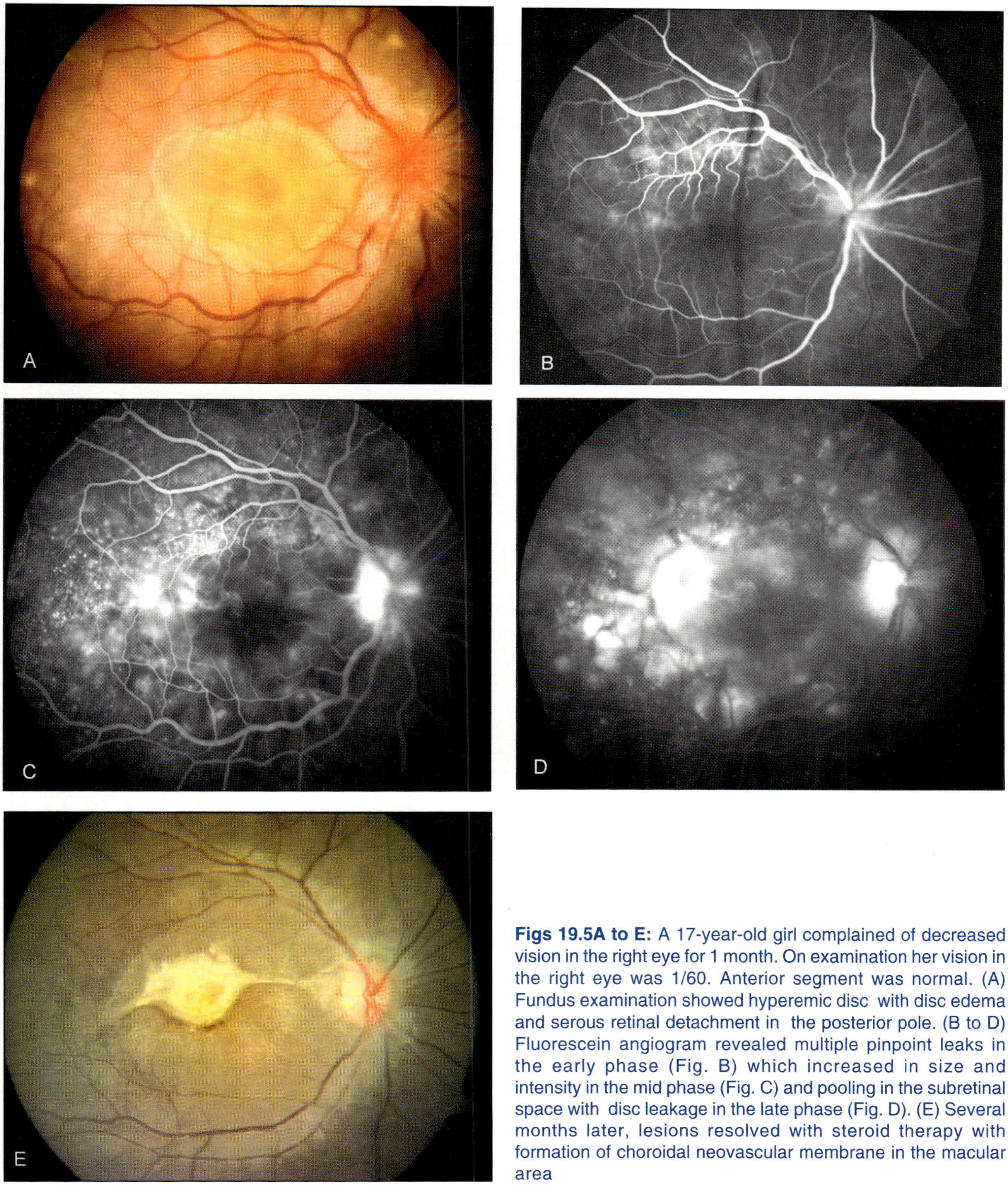

Figs 19.5A to E: A 17-year-old girl complained of decreased vision in the right eye for 1 month. On examination her vision in the right eye was 1/60. Anterior segment was normal. (A) Fundus examination showed hyperemic disc with disc edema and serous retinal detachment in the posterior pole. (B to D) Fluorescein angiogram revealed multiple pinpoint leaks in the early phase (Fig. B) which increased in size and intensity in the mid phase (Fig. C) and pooling in the subretinal space with disc leakage in the late phase (Fig. D). (E) Several months later, lesions resolved with steroid therapy with formation of choroidal neovascular membrane in the macular area

Convalescent phase of VKH

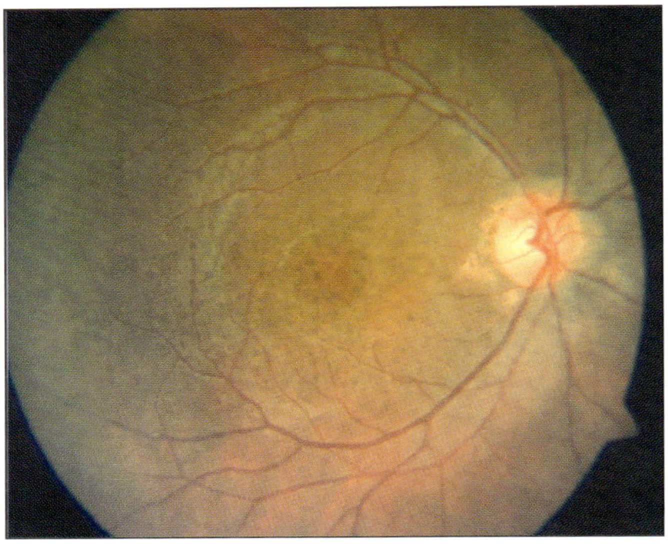

Fig. 19.6: Severe RPE atrophy in the chronic stage of VKH syndrome

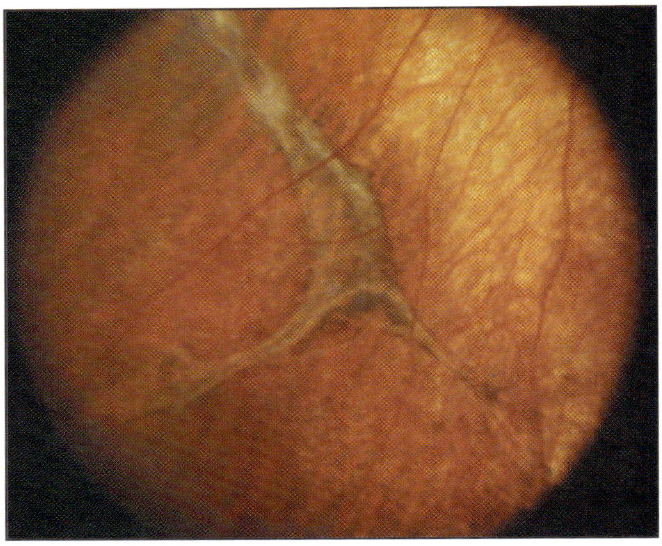

Fig. 19.7: Subretinal fibrosis in VKH syndrome

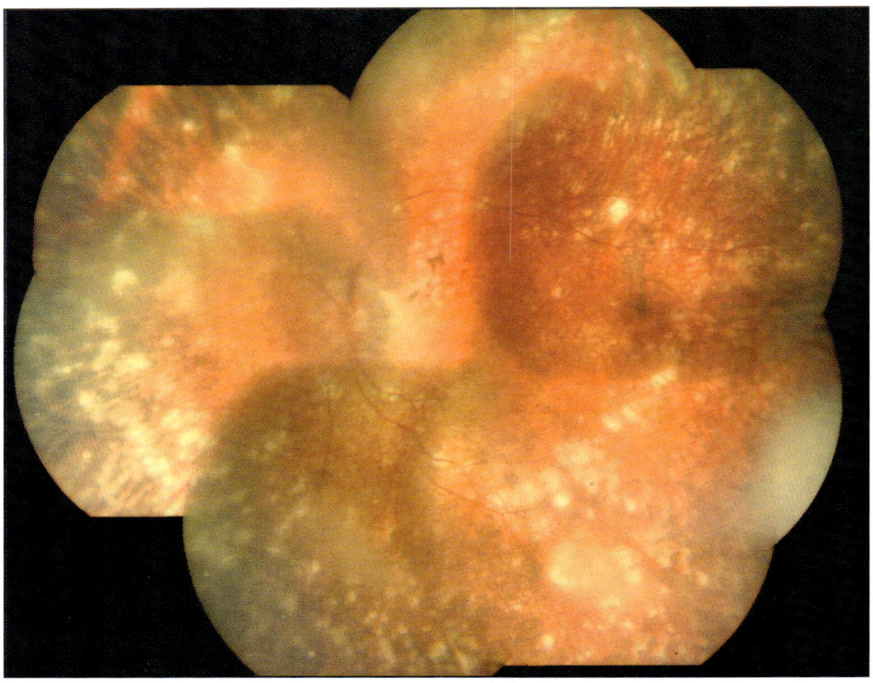

Fig. 19.8: Montage photograph showing the typical depigmented sunset glow fundus with characteristic yellow white Dalen-Fuchs' lesions in the periphery

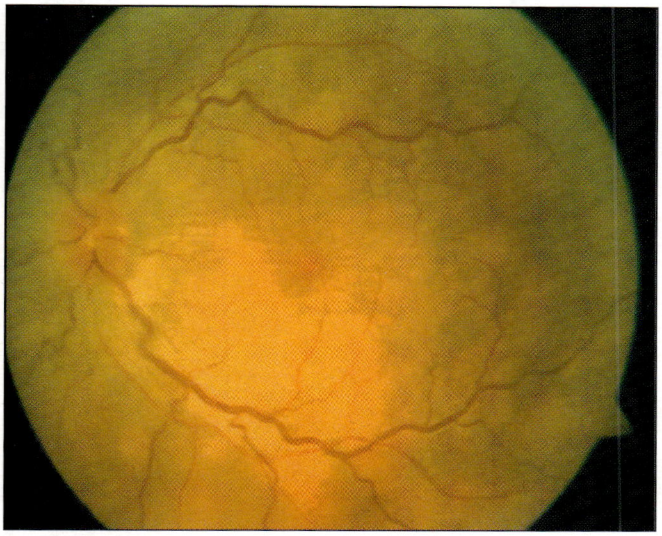

Fig. 19.9A: A 40-year-old man complained of sudden loss of vision in right eye for 1 week. Fundus examination showed optic disc edema, choroidal folds and exudative retinal detachment

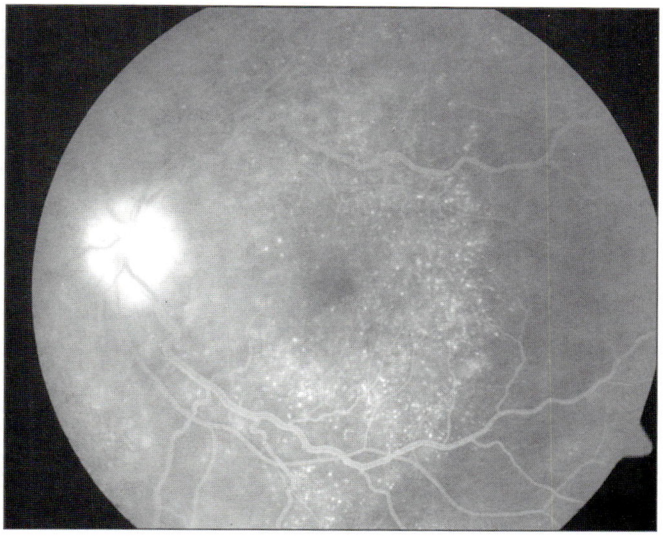

Fig. 19.9B: FFA of the same patient showing the classical starry sky appearance caused by hyperfluorescent dots at the level of retinal pigment epithelium along with disc leakage

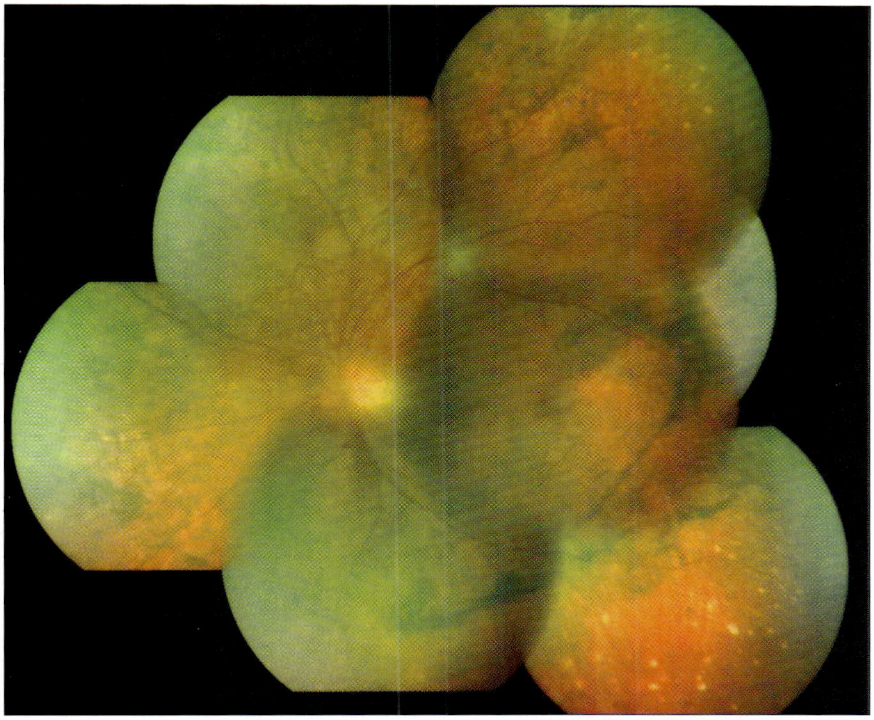

Fig. 19.10: Neovascularization of the disc in the convalescent phase of VKH syndrome

Systemic features in VKH Syndrome

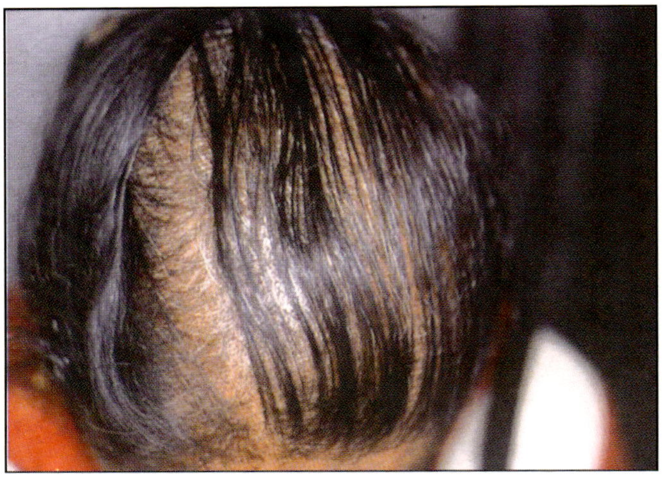

Fig. 19.11: Alopecia

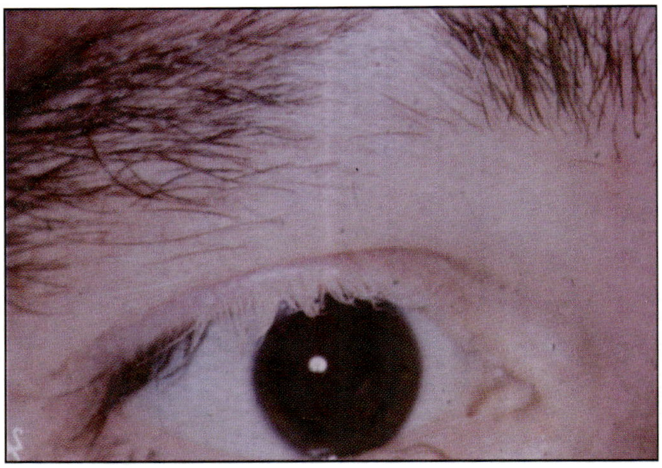

Fig. 19.12: Poliosis

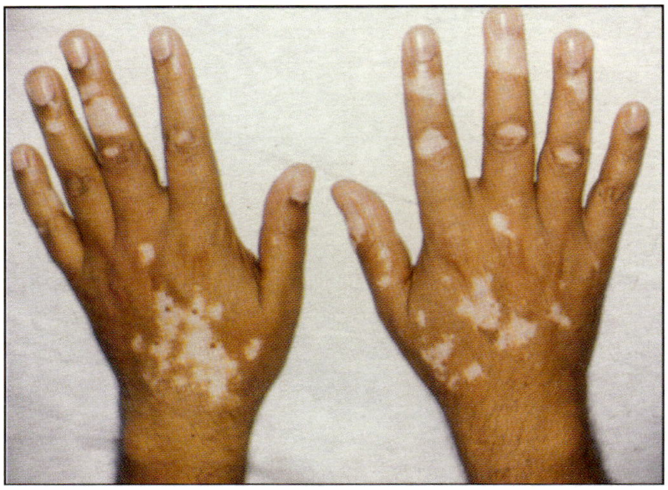

Fig. 19.13: Vitiligo

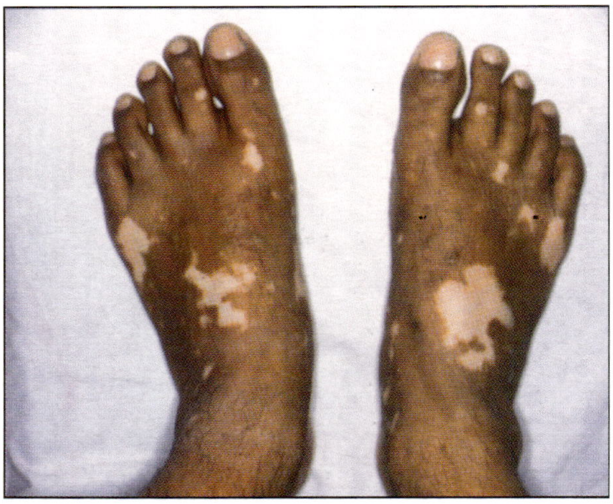

Fig. 19.14: Vitiligo

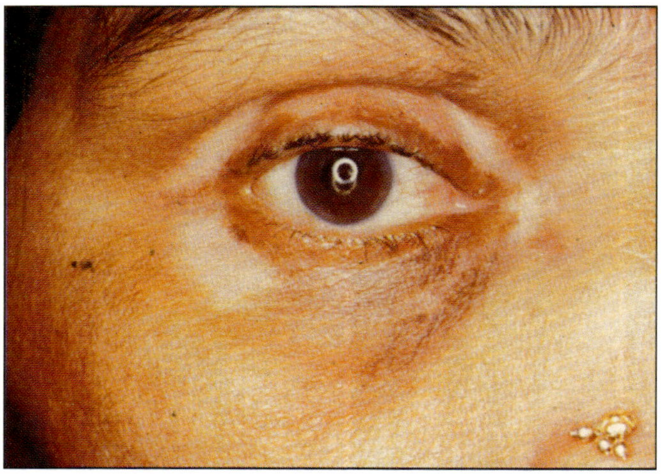

Fig. 19.15: Vitiligo

CHAPTER TWENTY

Sympathetic Ophthalmia

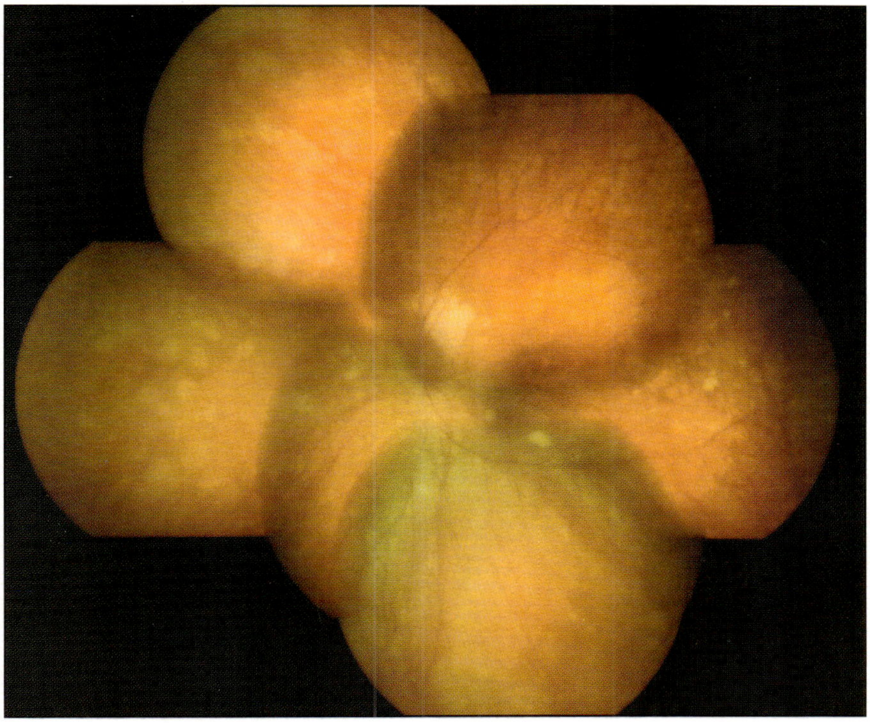

Sympathetic ophthalmia is a bilateral granulomatous panuveitis that occurs after either surgery or penetrating trauma to one eye. The incidence ranges from 0.19 to 0.7% in penetrating injuries and 0.007 to 0.015% in postsurgical patients. It is seen more commonly in men. The onset of inflammation is between 2 weeks and 3 months but cases have been reported as early as 5 days and as late as 66 years.

Ocular Features

Anterior segment: Granulomatous iridocyclitis with mutton fat keratic precipitates, anterior chamber cells and flare, and vitreous cells.

Posterior segment: Papillitis, exudative retinal detachment, focal elevated yellow—white choroidal infiltrates (Dalen-Fuchs' nodules) in the midperiphery, optic atrophy, subretinal fibrosis, choroidal atrophy.

Systemic Features

Alopecia, vitiligo, poliosis, dysacusis and cerebrospinal pleocytosis.

Investigations

FFA: Multiple areas of pin-point hyperfluorescence and in early phase at the level of retinal pigment epithelium and late pooling of dye in subretinal space.

Ultrasound: Marked choroidal thickening and serous retinal detachment

Treatment

- High-dose systemic corticosteroids along with topical and periocular steroids
- Immunosuppressives
- Role of enucleation is controversial.

REFERENCES

1. Rao NA: Sympathetic ophthalmia. In: Ryan SJ (Ed): Retina Medical retina St Louis, CV Mosby 1989;2:715-21.
2. Biswas J, Fogla R: Sympathetic ophthalmia following cyclo-cryotherapy—Report of a case with histopathological correlation. Ophthalmic Surgery and Laser 1996; 27:1305-08.
3. Biswas J: Neovascularisation of optic disc (NVD) in a case of sympathetic ophthalmia (SO). Uveitis Today (Proceedings of the Fourth International Symposium on Uveitis, Yokohama, Japan, 10-14 October, 1997) 1998;203-05.
4. Chu DS, Foster CS. Sympathetic ophthalmia. Int Ophthalmol Clin. 2002;42:179-85.
5. Ganesh SK, Narayana KM, Biswas J. Peripapillary choroidal atrophy in sympathetic ophthalmia and management with triple agent immunosuppression. Ocul Immunol Inflamm. 2003;11:61-65.

Clinical features of Sympathetic Ophthalmia

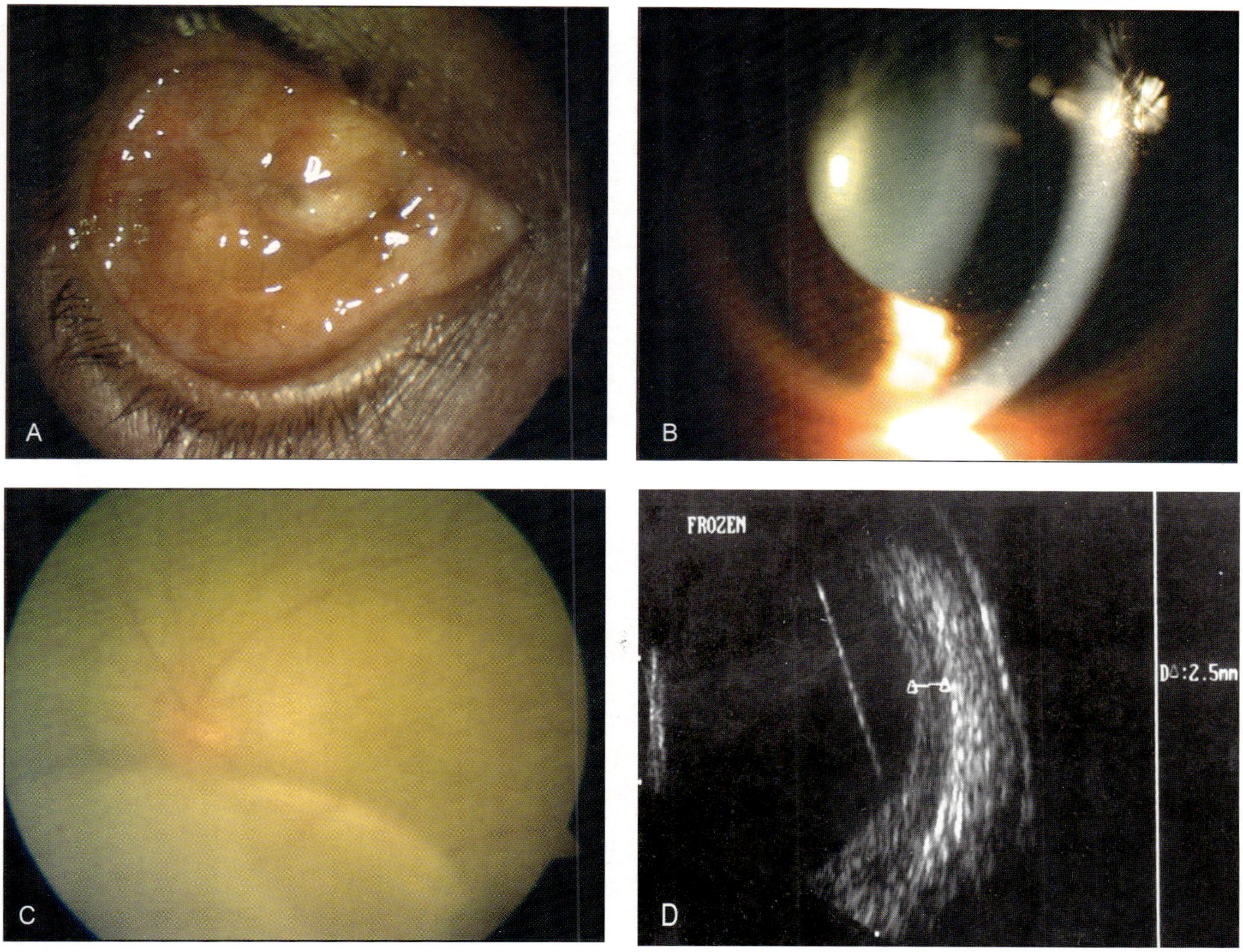

Figs 20.1A to D:

A. A 55-year-old lady complained of sudden onset of decreased vision in her left eye. She gave a history of penetrating injury in the right eye 5-year back following which enucleation was done

B. Slit lamp examination showed granulomatous anterior uveitis with mutton fat keratic precipitates

C. Fundus showed disc edema with exudative retinal detachment

D. Ultrasound examination revealed marked choroidal thickening confirming the diagnosis of sympathetic ophthalmia

Complications of Sympathetic Ophthalmia

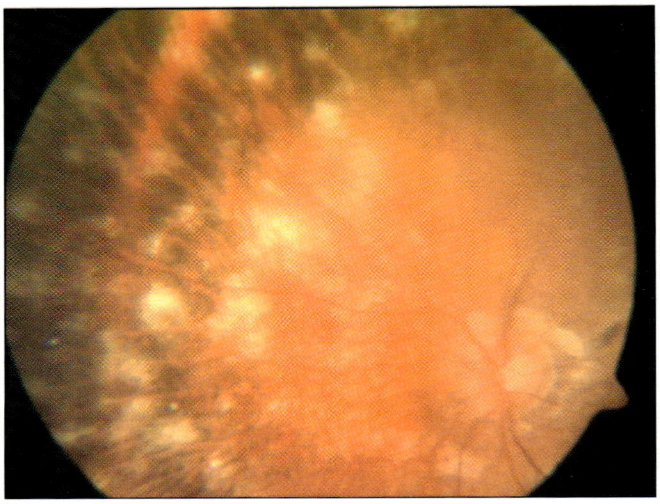

Fig. 20.2: Fundus photograph shows depigmented retina and Dalen-Fuchs nodules

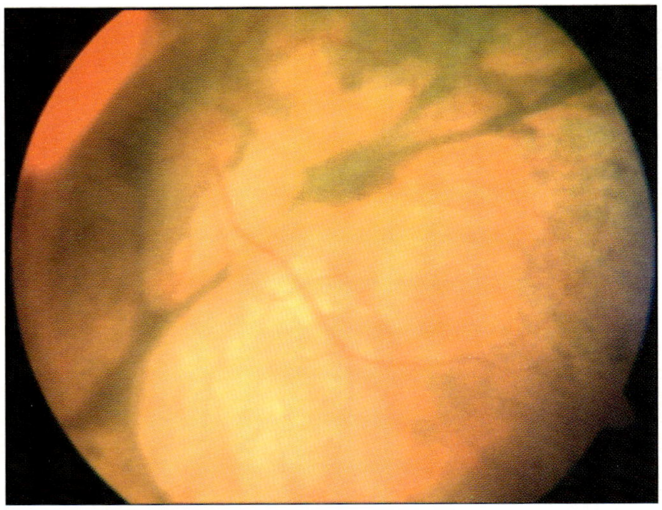

Fig. 20.3: Subretinal fibrosis and pigmentary alterations in a patient with sympathetic ophthalmia

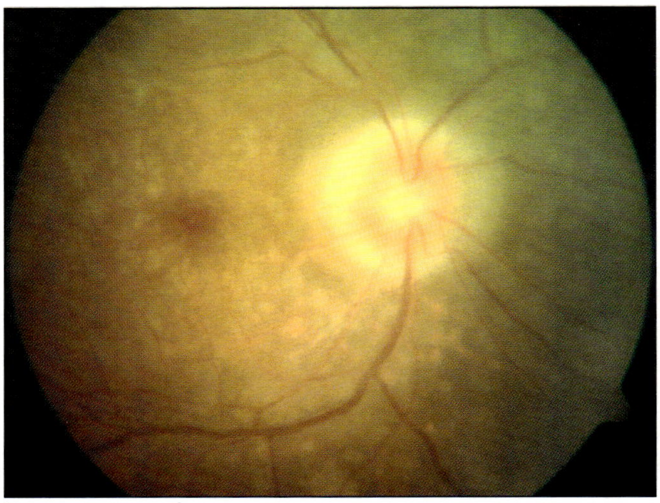

Fig. 20.4: Peripapillary atrophy in a case of resolved Sympathetic ophthalmia

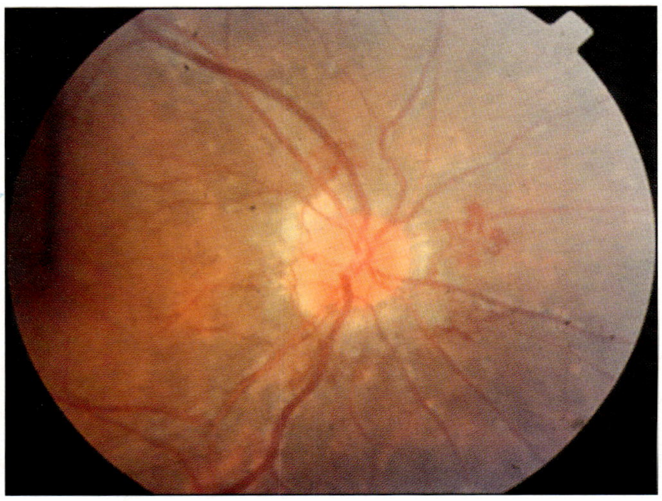

Fig. 20.5: Optic disc neovascularization complicating Sympathetic ophthalmia

Systemic Manifestations in Sympathetic Ophthalmia

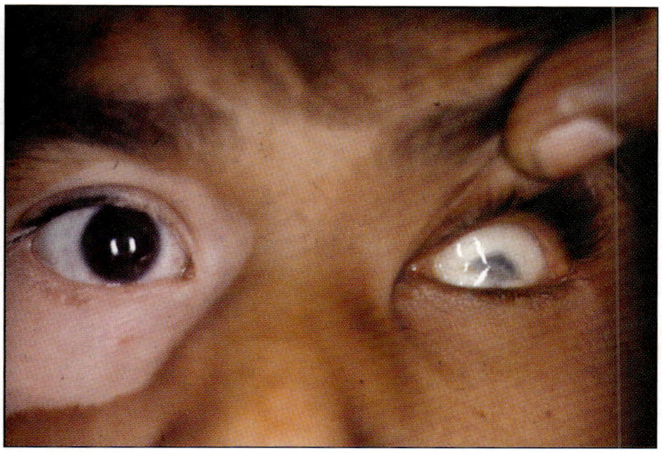

Fig. 20.6: Vitiligo in a patient with sympathetic ophthalmia

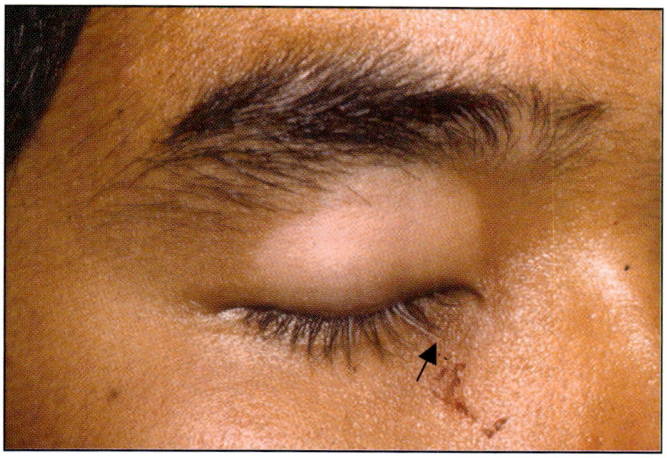

Fig. 20.7: Poliosis (arrow) in the same patient

CHAPTER TWENTY ONE

Behcet's Disease

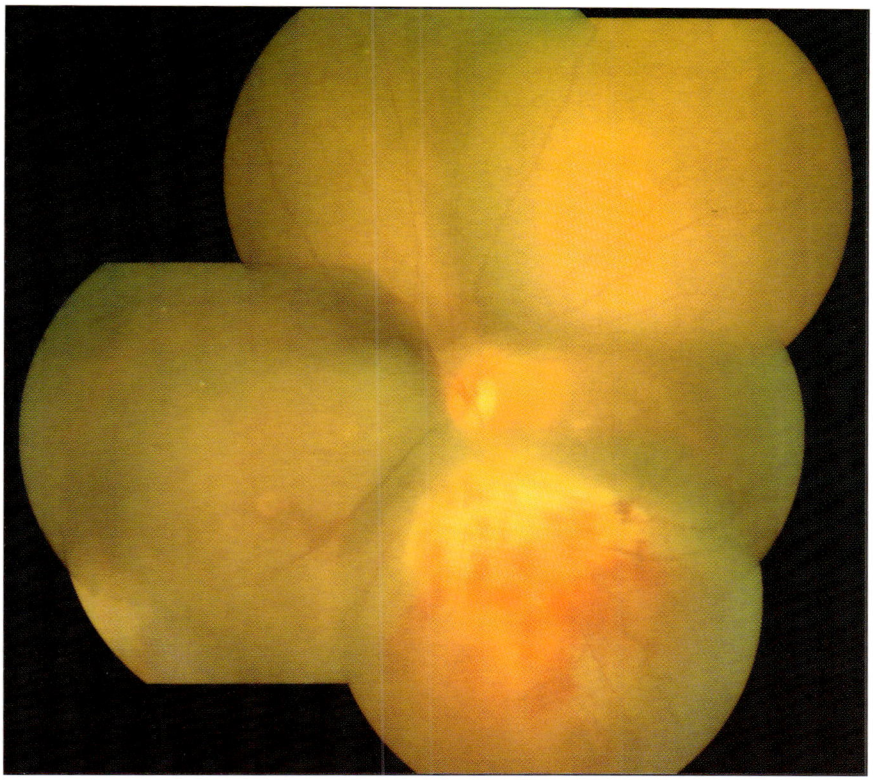

Systemic Features of Behcet's Disease

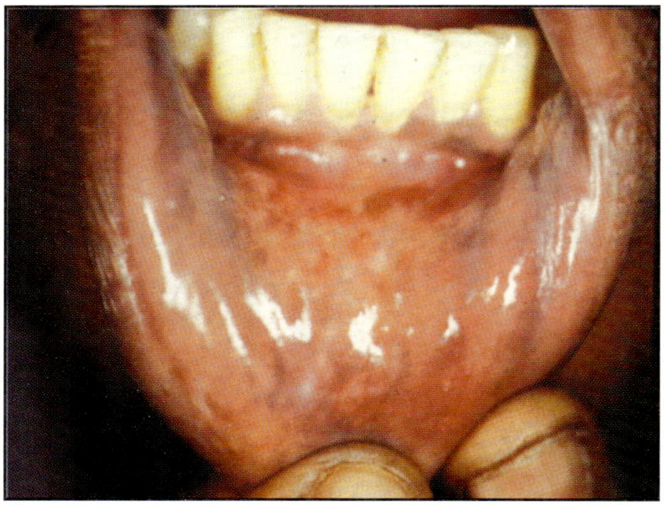

Fig. 21.4: Aphthous ulcers involving the gums and buccal mucosa in Behcet's disease

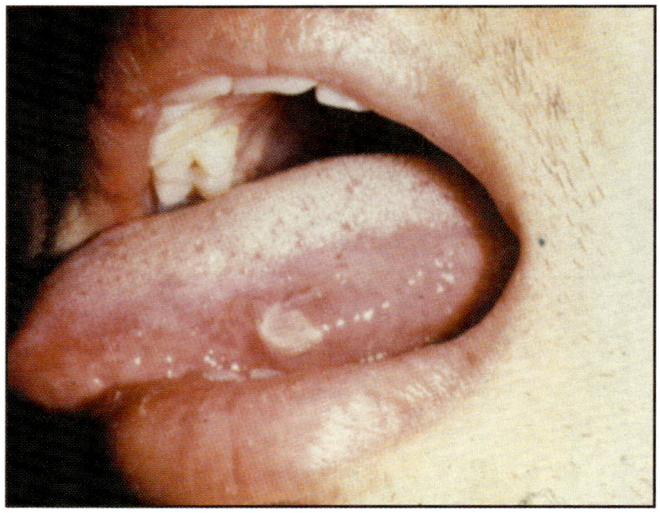

Fig. 21.5: Large ulcer on the under surface of the tongue

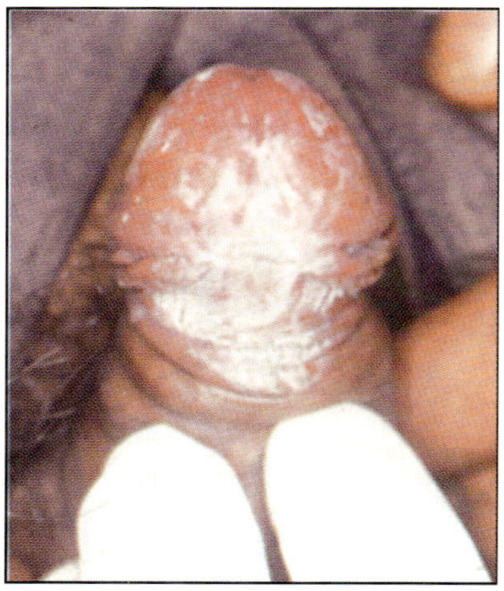

Fig. 21.6: Penile ulcer in Behcet's disease

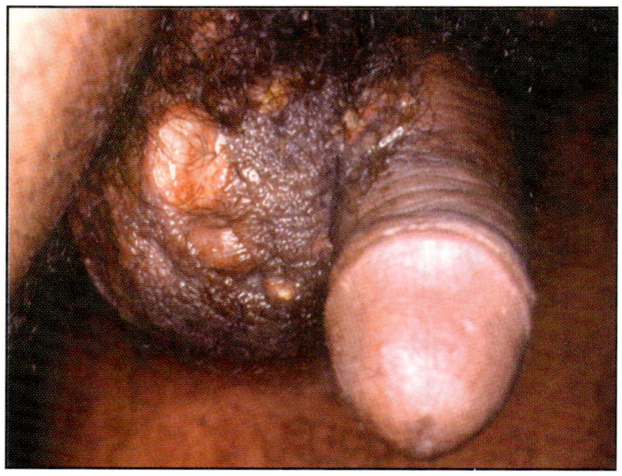

Fig. 21.7: Scrotal ulcer in Behcet's disease

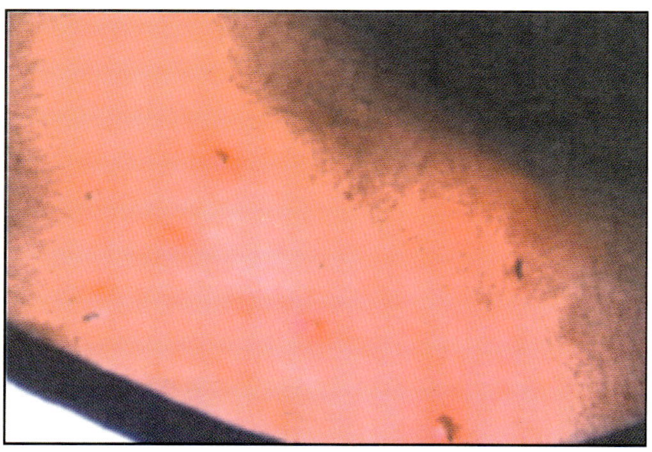

Fig. 21.8: Erythema nodosum like lesions on the anterior surface of the leg in a patient with Behcet's disease

CHAPTER TWENTY TWO

Tuberculosis

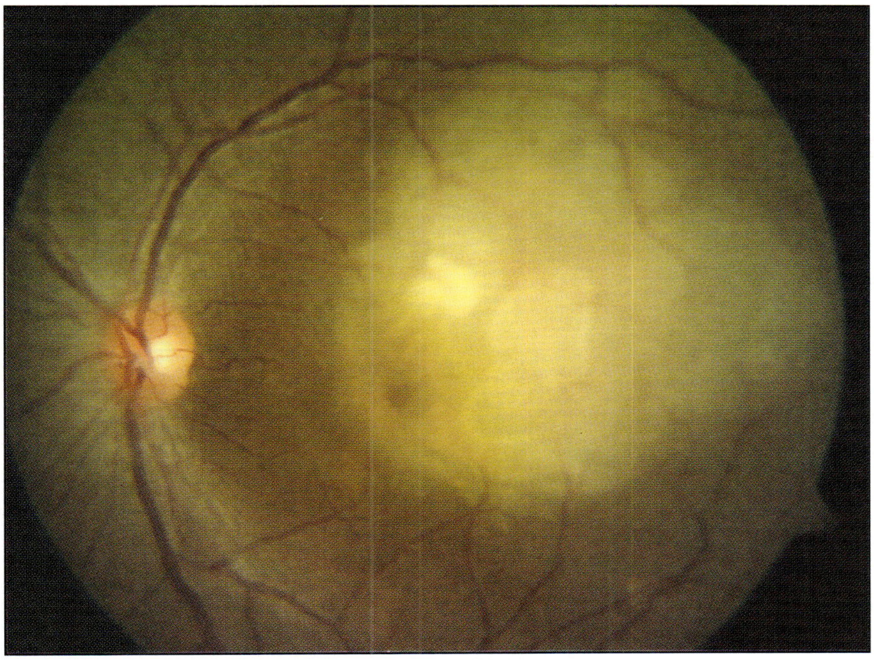

Tuberculosis, caused by *Mycobacterium tuberculosis* is increasing recently due to the AIDS epidemic. The disease becomes active in only 10 percent of infected individuals. Ocular tuberculosis can be divided into two types—primary and secondary.

Primary: The organism infects the eye primarily and involves the conjunctiva, cornea and sclera.

Secondary: Ocular involvement occurs secondary to hematogenous spread and presents as tubercular uveitis.

Ocular Features

Anterior segment: Conjunctivitis, keratitis, scleritis, granulomatous uveitis

Posterior segment: Most common manifestation is choroiditis/subretinal TB abscess.

Disseminated choroiditis—Discrete yellow, white or gray choroidal tubercles, 0.5-3 mm in diameter more common in posterior pole, associated with disc edema and retinal hemorrhages.

Focal choroiditis—Presents as a single choroidal tubercle about 2 to 3 disc diameters in size with overlying serous retinal detachment.

Other manifestations include, retinal vasculitis, optic neuritis, and panophthalmitis.

Systemic Associations

Tuberculosis of lungs, spine, gastrointestinal tract, brain or miliary TB.

Investigations

1. Total white cell count with differential count
2. Erythrocyte sedimentation rate
3. Tuberculin skin test (Mantoux test)
4. Chest X-ray/CT chest
5. Aqueous aspirate/vitreous biopsy can be done for acid fast bacilli stain, culture and polymerase chain reaction in cases of diagnostic dilemmas.
6. Ultrasound B scan which shows a hyperechoic mass with absence of scleral echo in cases of subretinal abscess.
7. Fundus fluorescein angiography in cases of choroiditis shows early hypofluorescence with hyperfluorescence in late stages.

Treatment

1. Antitubercular therapy including isoniazid, rifampicin, pyrazinamide, ethambutol and streptomycin under care of an internist (3-4 drug therapy)
2. Low dose oral corticosteroids

REFERENCES

1. Helm CJ, Holland GN. Ocular tuberculosis. Surv Ophthalmol 1993; 38:229-256.
2. Biswas J, Madhavan HN, Gopal L, Badrinath S. Intraocular tuberculosis. Clinicopathologic study of five cases. Retina 1995;15: 461-468.
3. Biswas J, Badrinath S. Ocular morbidity in patients with active systemic tuberculosis. Int Ophthalmol 1996;19:293-298.

Tubercular Choroiditis

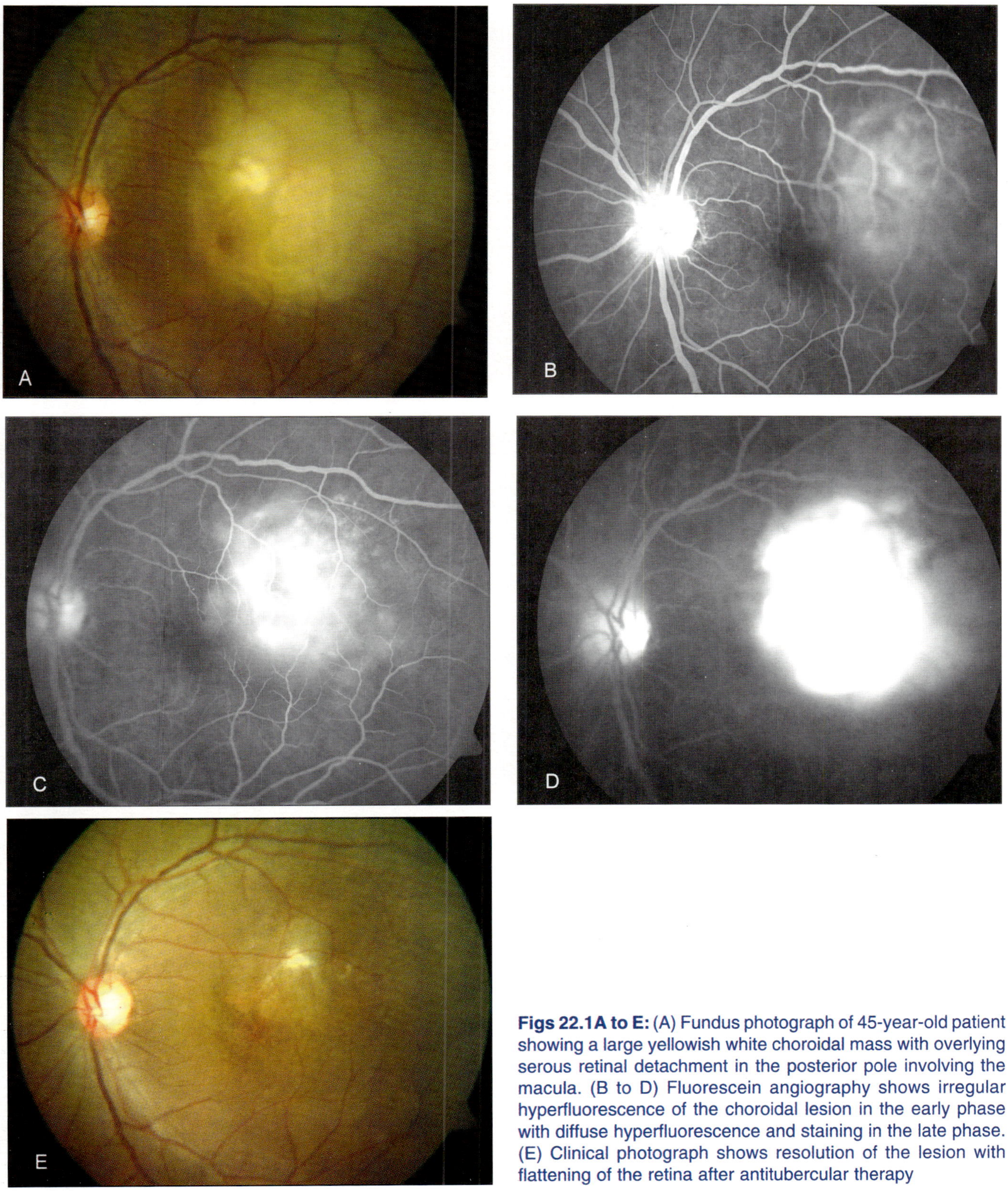

Figs 22.1A to E: (A) Fundus photograph of 45-year-old patient showing a large yellowish white choroidal mass with overlying serous retinal detachment in the posterior pole involving the macula. (B to D) Fluorescein angiography shows irregular hyperfluorescence of the choroidal lesion in the early phase with diffuse hyperfluorescence and staining in the late phase. (E) Clinical photograph shows resolution of the lesion with flattening of the retina after antitubercular therapy

Miliary Tuberculosis

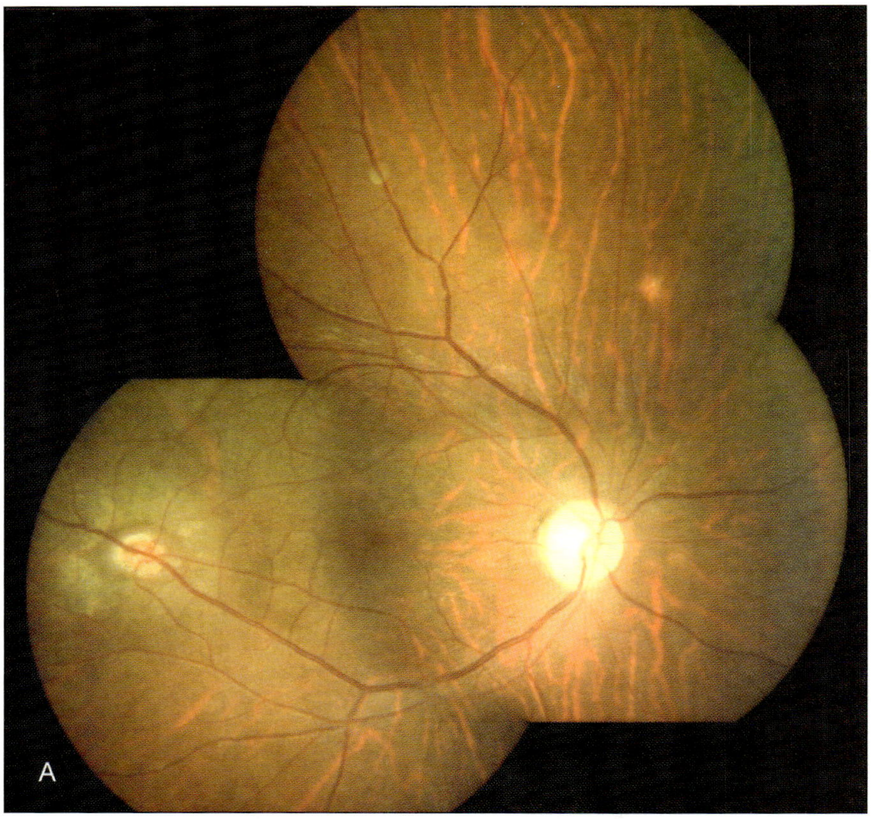

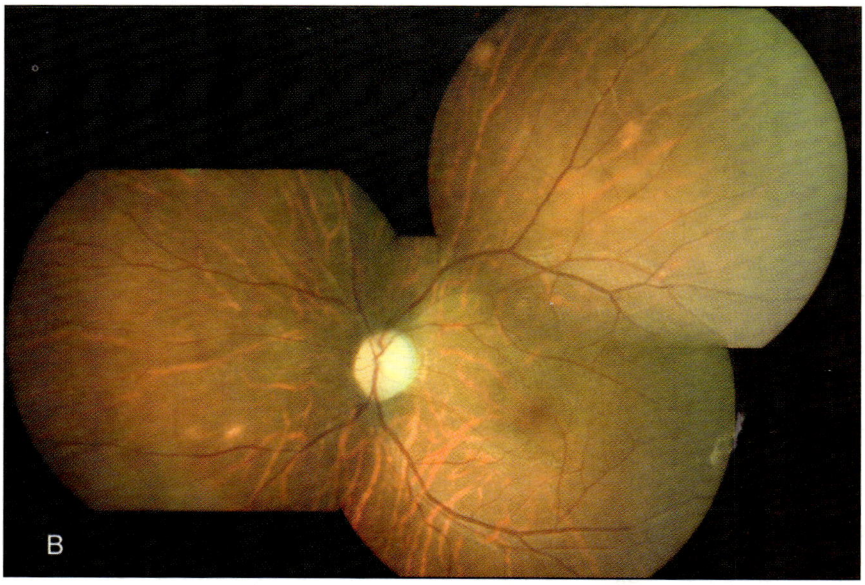

Figs 22.2A and B: Fundus photograph of the right and left eyes of an 18-year-old patient with miliary tuberculosis showing bilateral optic atrophy with patches of resolving choroiditis. MRI of brain showed multiple tuberculomas and chest X-ray revealed bilateral pulmonary TB

Subretinal Abscess due to Tuberculosis

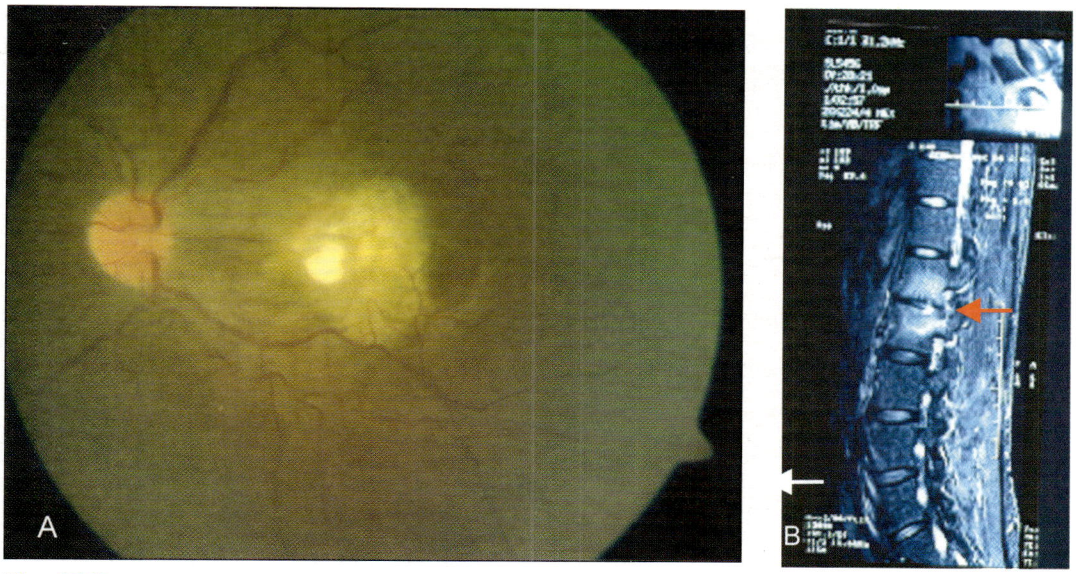

Figs 22.3:

A. Fundus photograph of a 32-year-old patient showing subretinal abscess with ILM folds over the macular area. PCR test of aqueous aspirate was positive for *Mycobacterium tuberculosis.* Chest X-ray showed fibrotic lesions in the left lower zone of the lung.

B. MRI spine showed heterogenous signals from L1-L2 vertebrae with loss of intervening intervertebral disc morphology and breach of upper end plate area of L2 which was suggestive of Pott's spine (→)

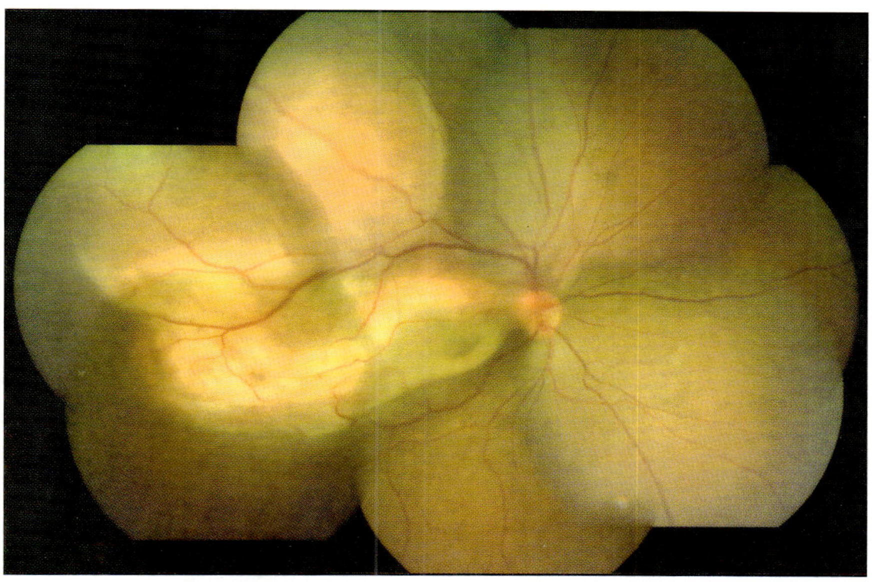

Fig. 22.4: Fundus photograph of a 14-year-old girl with systemic tuberculosis showing large subretinal abscess with overlying retinal detachment

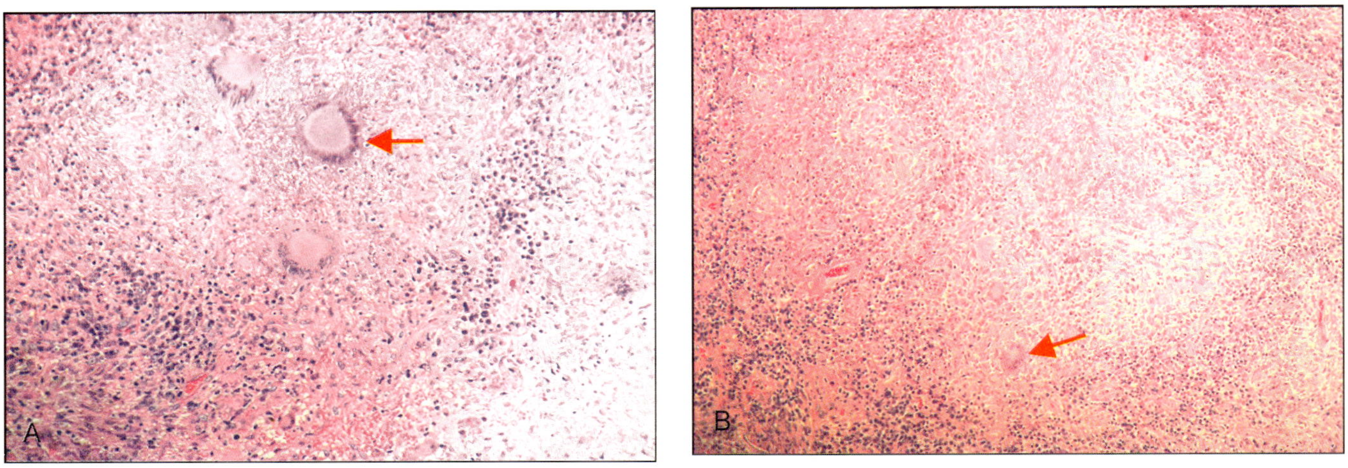

Figs 22.8A and B: Duodenal biopsy revealed granulomatous inflammation with areas of caseating necrosis consistent with intestinal tuberculosis (arrow)

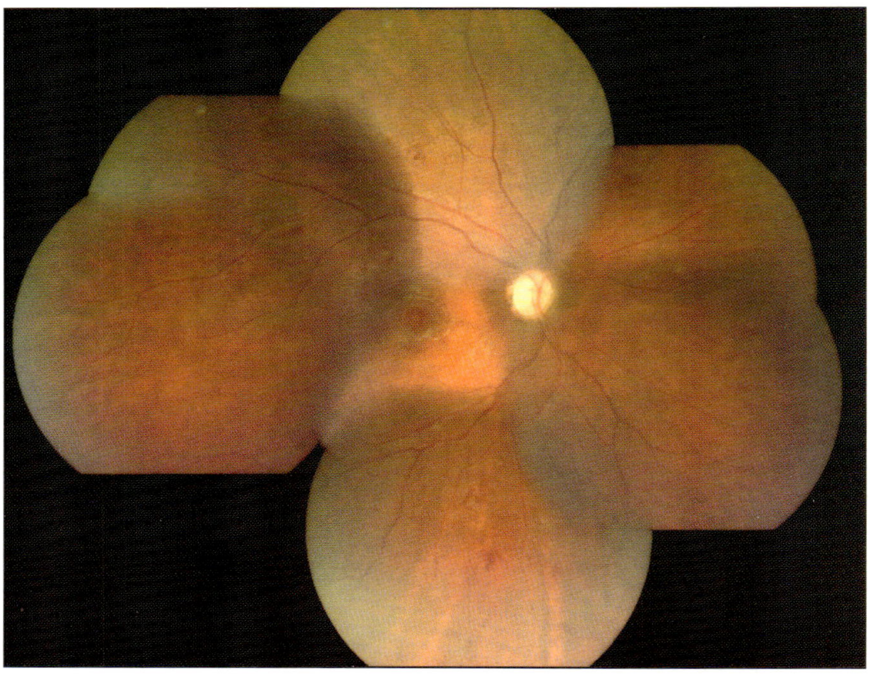

Fig. 22.9: Fundus photograph of the right eye following antitubercular therapy and corticosteroids. Vision recovered to 6/36 in both eyes at the end of six months of treatment

Complications of TB Choroiditis

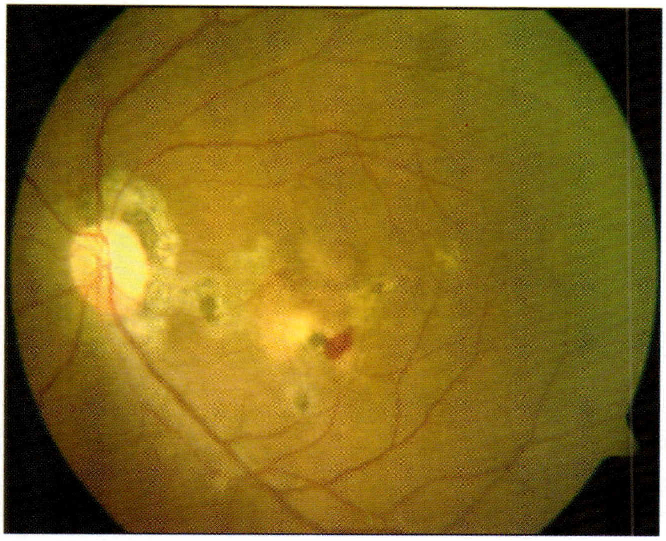

Fig. 22.10A: Fundus photograph showing subfoveal neovascular membrane in a patient with healed tubercular choroiditis

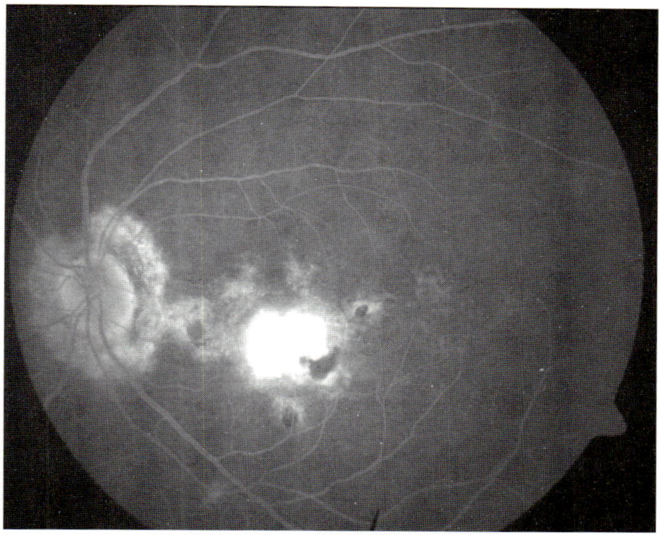

Fig. 22.10B: Fluorescein angiogram shows hyperfluorescence due to leakage in the late phase

Section 5
Infectious Uveitis

CHAPTER TWENTY THREE

Endogenous Endophthalmitis

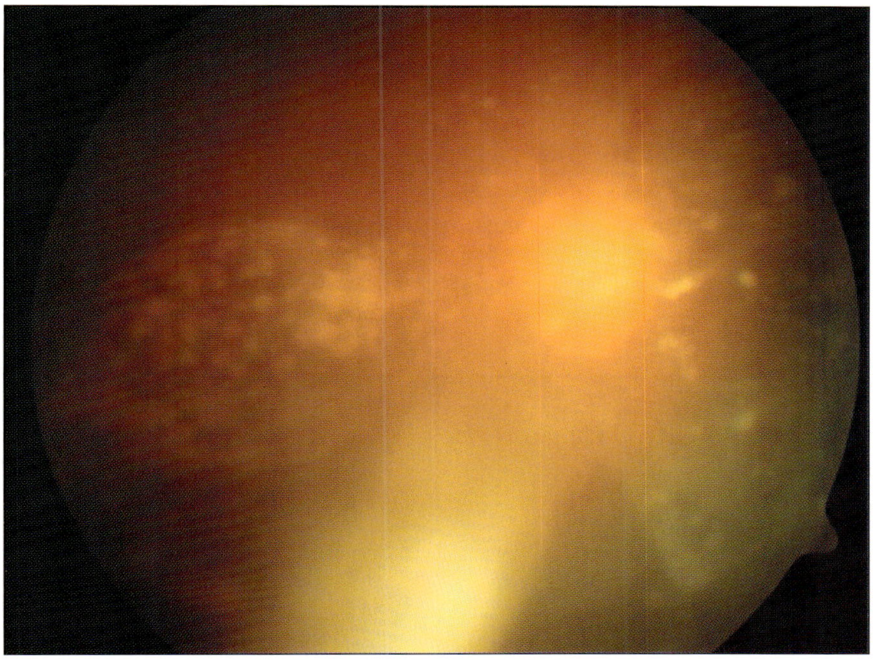

Section 6
Systemic Diseases associated with Uveitis

CHAPTER TWENTY FOUR

Systemic Diseases associated with Uveitis

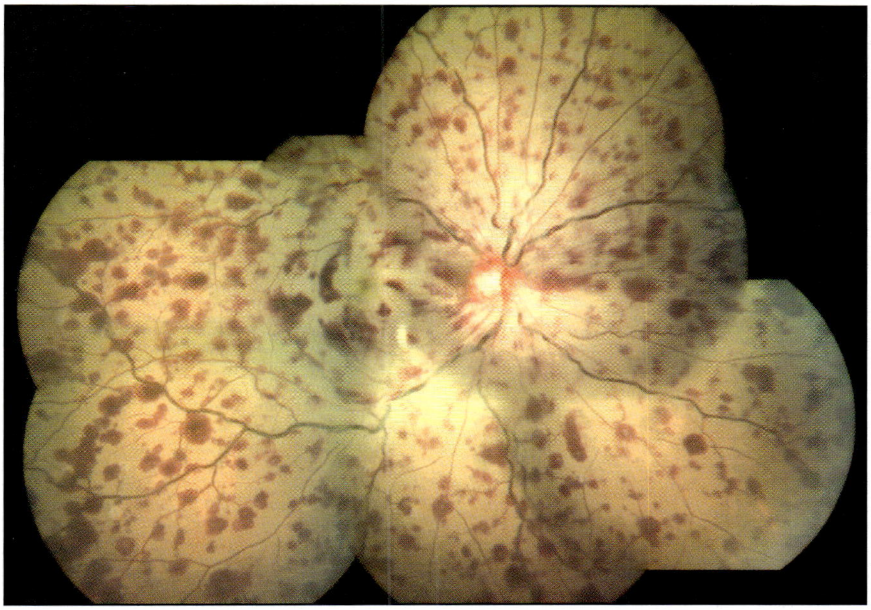

Systemic diseases associated with uveitis can be autoimmune or infectious in origin.

Autoimmune: Sarcoidosis, collagen vascular diseases, seronegative spondyloarthropathies, gout, multiple sclerosis.

Infection: Tuberculosis, leprosy, syphilis, AIDS.

WEGENER'S GRANULOMATOSIS

Wegener's granulomatosis is characterized by granulomatous necrotizing vasculitis of upper and lower respiratory tracts along with renal involvement. Ocular involvement is seen in 50 percent cases. It is seen in fourth and fifth decades of life.

Ocular Features

Conjunctivitis, episcleritis, scleritis, peripheral ulcerative keratitis, anterior, intermediate or posterior uveitis, vitreous hemorrhage, central retinal artery and venous occlusion.

Systemic Features

Fever, malaise, weight loss, arthralgias, myalgias, sinus pain, epistaxis, otitis media, cough, hemoptysis, dyspnea, pleural effusion, proteinuria, hematuria, red blood cell casts, renal insufficiency, purpuric skin rashes, peripheral and cranial neuropathies, seizures, stroke.

Investigations

Complete blood count, erythrocyte sedimentation rate, C reactive protein, rheumatoid factor, antinuclear body, antineutrophil cytoplasmic antibody (cytoplasmic pattern)—c-ANCA, Urine routine.

Treatment

- Corticosteroids
- Immunosuppressives—cyclophosphamide, azathioprine, methotrexate.

SYSTEMIC LUPUS ERYTHEMATOSUS

Systemic lupus erythematosus (SLE) is an autoimmune disease characterized by arthritis, glomerulonephritis, dermatitis, and various hematological and neurological manifestations. It is seen in 80 percent females especially in the child bearing age.

Ocular Features

Episcleritis, scleritis, keratoconjunctivitis sicca, uveitis, lupus retinopathy—Cotton-wool spots, retinal hemorrhages, microaneurysms, retinal arterial or venous occlusion, neovascularization, vitreous hemorrhage, vasculitis, papilledema.

Systemic Features

Malar rash, discoid rash, photosensitivity, oral ulcers, arthritis, pleuritis, pericarditis, nephritis, seizures, psychosis, anemia, leucopenia, thrombocytopenia.

Investigations

- Complete blood count
- Erythrocyte sedimentation rate
- C-reactive protein
- Rheumatoid factor
- Antinuclear antibodies
- Antiphospholipid antibodies
- Urine routine.

Treatment

- Corticosteroids
- Immunosuppressives—Cyclophosphamide, azathioprine, methotrexate.

Wegener's Granulomatosis

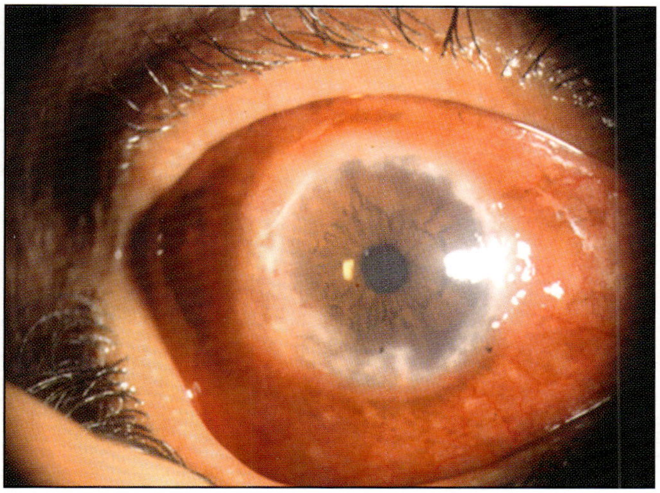

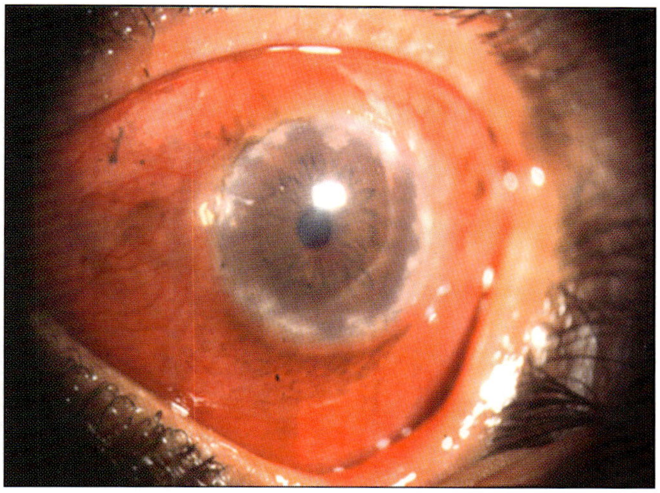

Figs 24.1 and 24.2: Slit lamp photograph of right and left eye showing diffuse necrotising scleritis and kerato uveitis in a patient with Wegener's granulomatosis

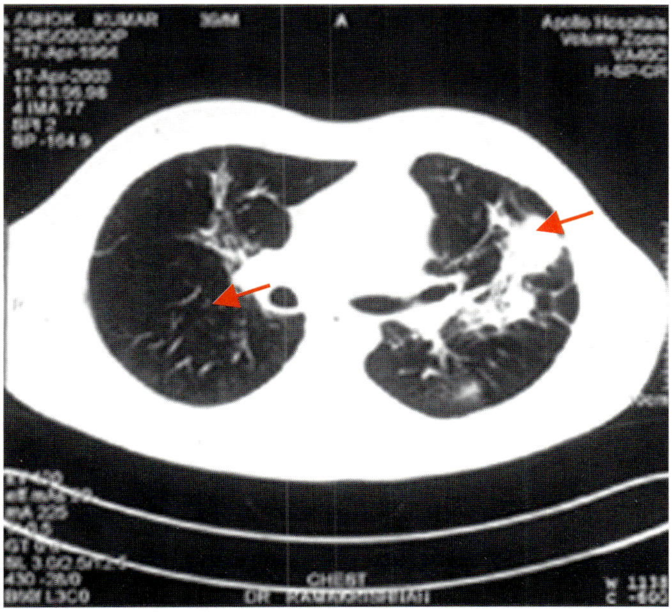

Fig. 24.3: CT chest of the same patient showing diffuse infiltrates and nodular lesions in the lungs suggestive of pulmonary involvement (arrow)

A 33-year-old man complained of pain, redness, photophobia in left eye for 4 months.

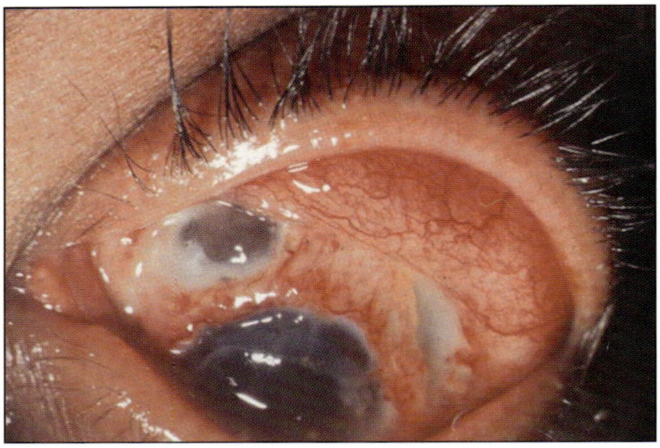

Fig. 24.4: Slit lamp photograph showing necrotizing scleritis with peripheral ulcerative keratitis. Area of uveal prolapse is also seen

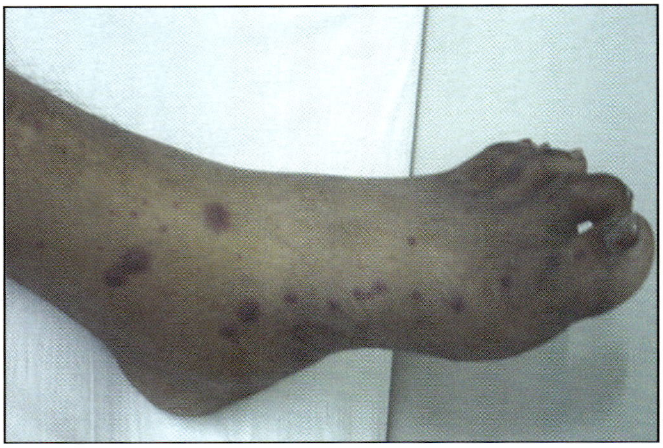

Fig. 24.5: External photograph showing palpable purpur spot

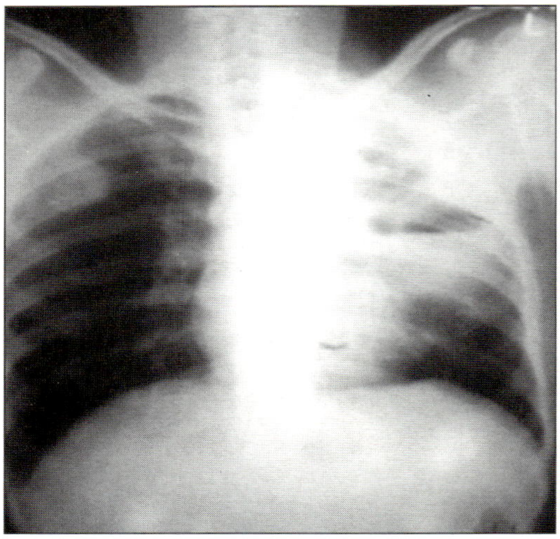

Fig. 24.6: Chest X-ray showing cavitatory lesion in right lung with pleural effusion in the left lung

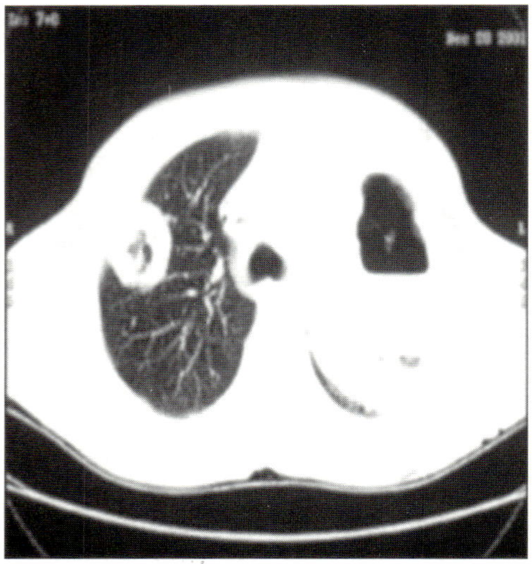

Fig. 24.7: CT scan showing cavities in both the lungs with pleural and pericardial effusion

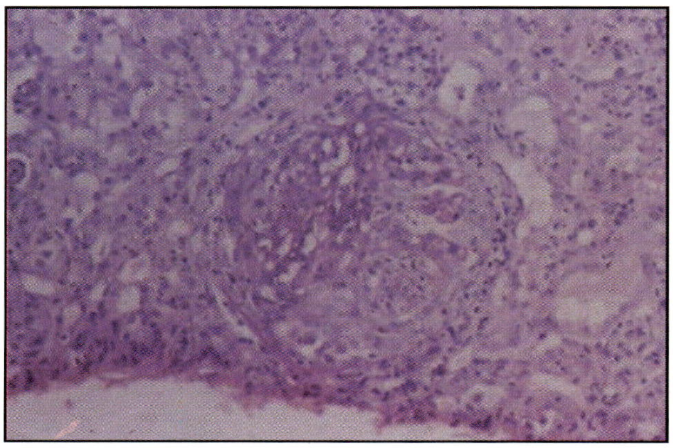

Fig. 24.8: HPE of renal biopsy revealing crescentric glomerulonephritis

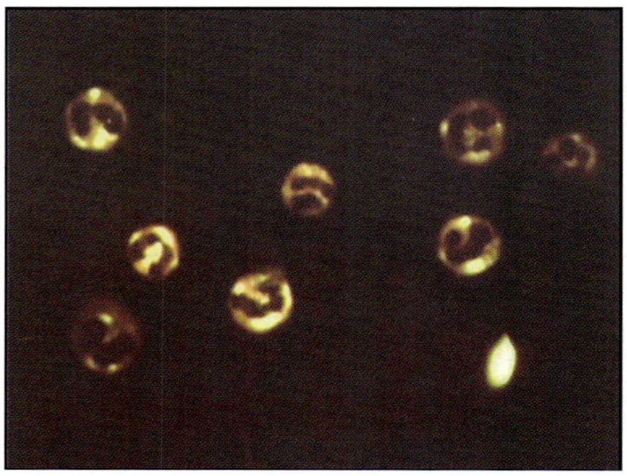

Fig. 24.9: Photomicrograph showing positive cANCA

Systemic Lupus Erythematosus (SLE)

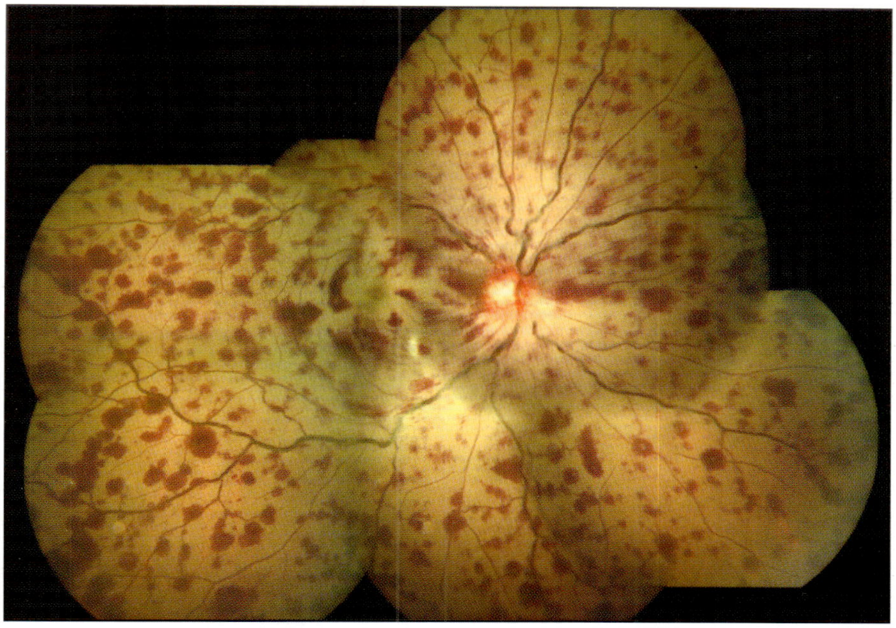

Fig. 24.10: A 29-year-old lady, a known case of SLE and scleroderma , complained of sudden painless loss of vision in right eye since 1 day. Raynaud's phenomenon was also positive for which amputation of two toes was done. She had a history of abortion 7-year back. Her vision in right and left eye was light perception and 6/6 respectively. Fundus photograph of the right eye shows a pale and edematous retina with multiple intraretinal hemorrhages and roth spots

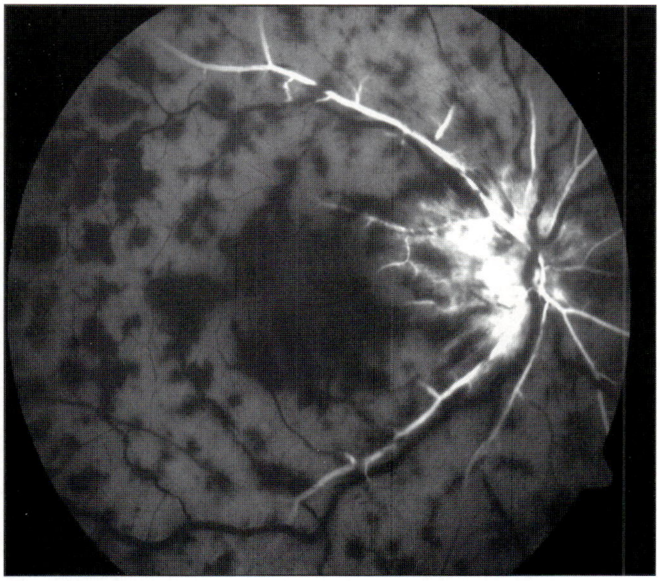

Fig. 24.11: Fluorescein angiogram shows blocked fluorescence due to retinal hemorrhages and central retinal artery and vein occlusion. Patient was diagnosed to have SLE

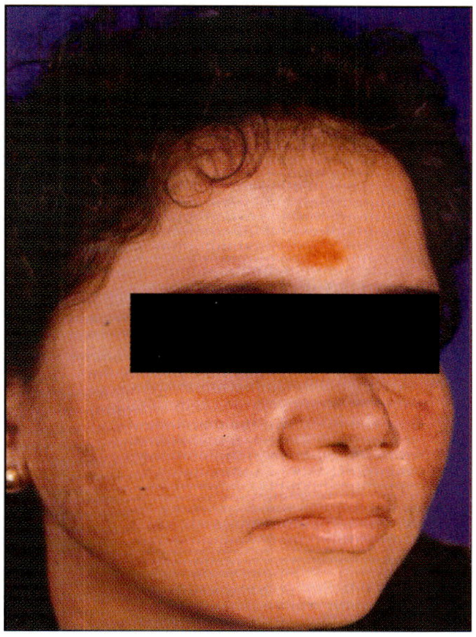

Fig. 24.12: Butterfly malar rash

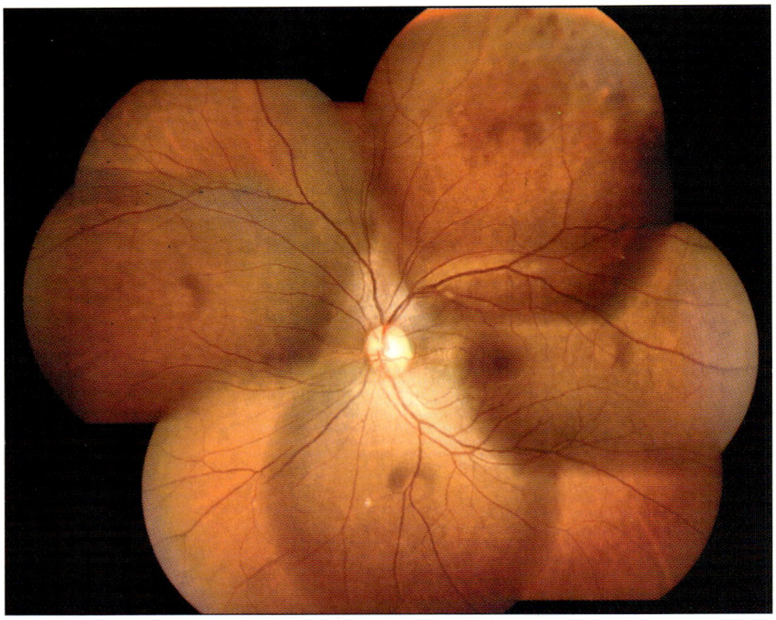

Fig. 24.13: Fundus photograph of the left eye shows sclerosed vessel and few retinal hemorrhages in superotemporal quadrant

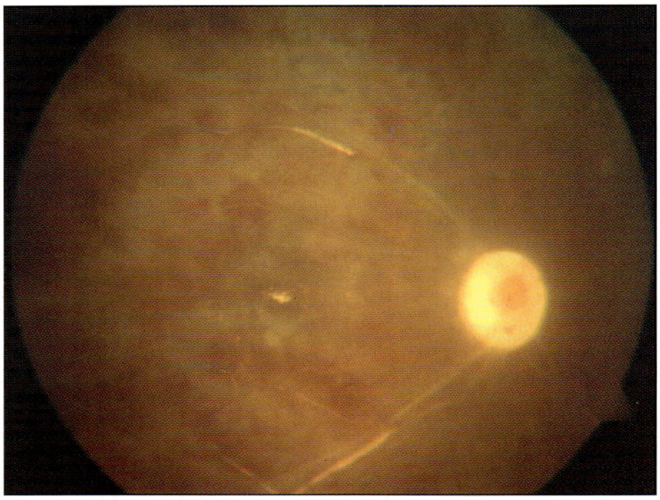

Fig. 24.14: Fundus photograph shows sclerosed vessels, and pale optic disc following treatment with immunosuppressives and steroids

Systemic Manifestations

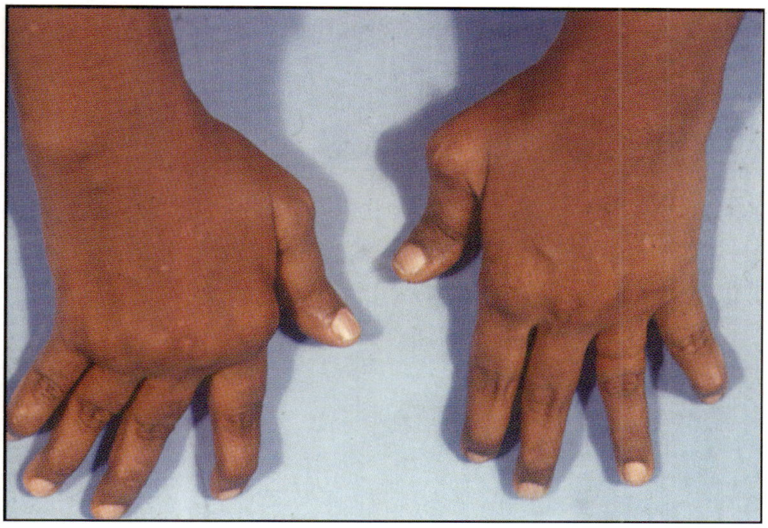

Fig. 24.15: Rheumatoid arthritis

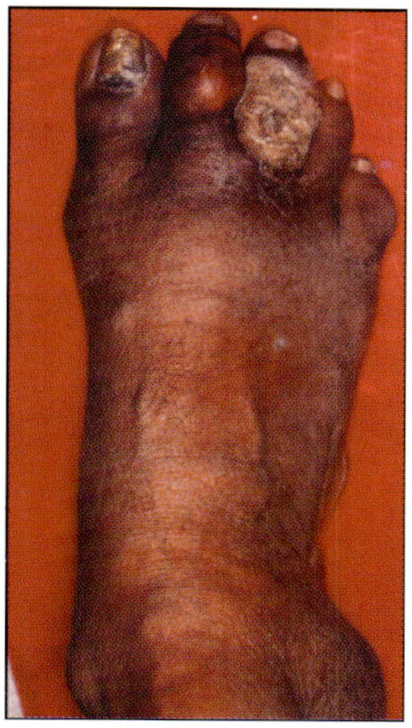

Fig. 24.16: Gout

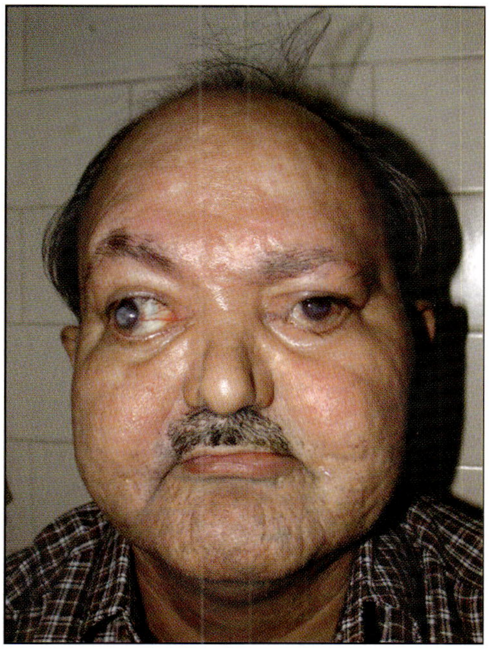

Fig. 24.17: Leprosy

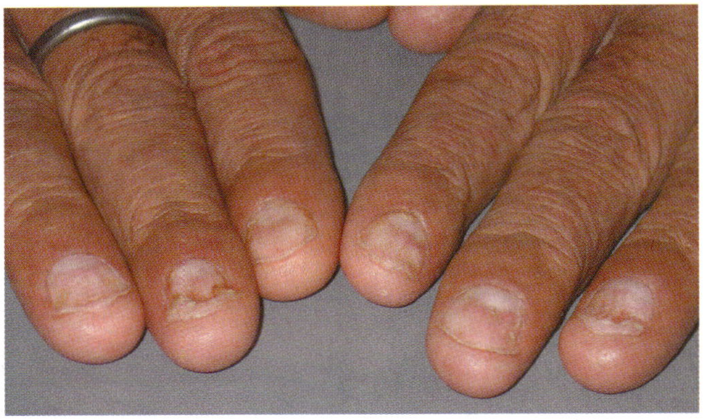

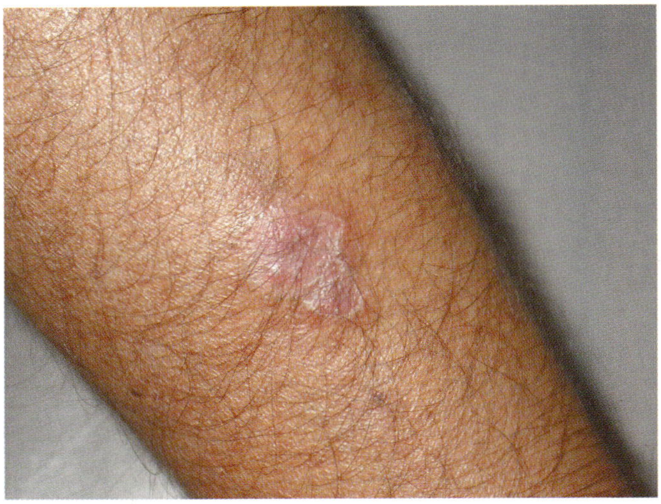

Figs 24.18A and B: Reiter's disease

Section 7
Complications of Uveitis

CHAPTER TWENTY FIVE

Complications of Uveitis

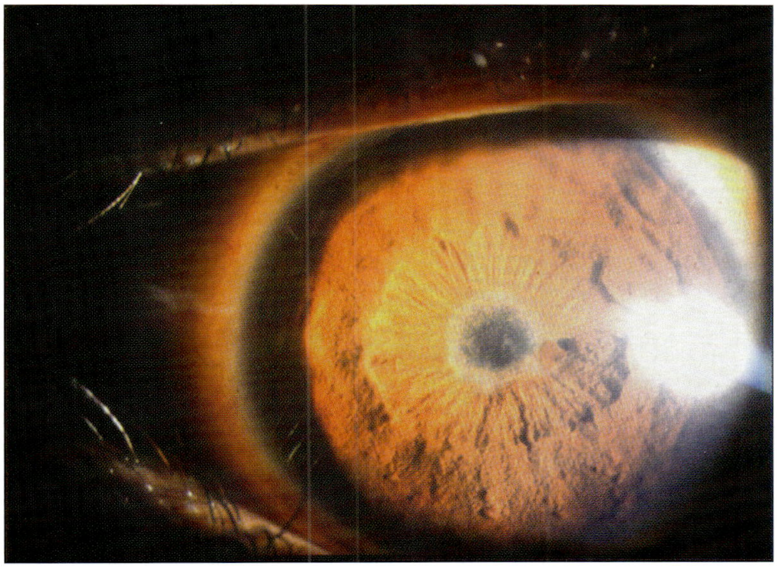

BAND SHAPED KERATOPATHY

Occurs due to deposition of calcium hydroxyapatite in the cornea at the level of Bowman's membrane and elevation of pH due to evaporation of tears. BSK occurs commonly in chronic uveitis specially juvenile idiopathic uveitis. It is chelated with disodium EDTA after removal of corneal epithelium.

CATARACT

Posterior subcapsular cataract is a frequent complication of uveitis due to recurrent inflammation and use of corticosteroid therapy. It occurs in 50 percent of patients with juvenile idiopathic arthritis, pars planitis and Fuchs' heterochromic iridocyclitis.

GLAUCOMA

It occurs in 25 percent of patients with uveitis. Various mechanisms include blockage of trabecular meshwork by inflammatory cells, trabeculitis, peripheral synechiae formation, posterior synechiae formation with iris bombe and pupillary block, secondary angle closure due to ciliary body edema and serous retinal detachment. Corticosteroid induced raised intraocular pressure is also one of the major cause of glaucoma in uveitis.

CYSTOID MACULAR EDEMA

It is the one of the most common complications seen in uveitis especially in intermediate uveitis. Breakdown of blood retinal barrier occurs due to the release of inflammatory mediators, i. e. cytokines, arachidonic acid metabolites and oxygen free radicals in the vitreous, this causes the leakage from the perifoveal capillaries resulting in cystoid macular edema.

HYPOTONY

It is a rare and serious complication of chronic uveitis that results from decreased aqueous secretion from an atrophic or fibrotic ciliary body, increased aqueous outflow from disrupted uveoscleral pathways and ciliary body detachment by cyclitic membrane formation. The sequelae of hypotony may be keratopathy with descemets folds, optic disc edema, maculopathy, and phthisis bulbi.

RETINAL DETACHMENT

- Rhegmatogenous retinal detachment—Acute retinal necrosis, *Cytomegalovirus retinitis*
- Tractional retinal detachment—Pars planitis

OTHER COMPLICATIONS

- Vitreous hemorrhage
- Disc neovascularization
- Choroidal neovascular membrane
- Subretinal fibrosis
- Steroid induced central serous retinopathy
- Neuroretinitis
- Macular hole

Anterior Segment Complications in Uveitis

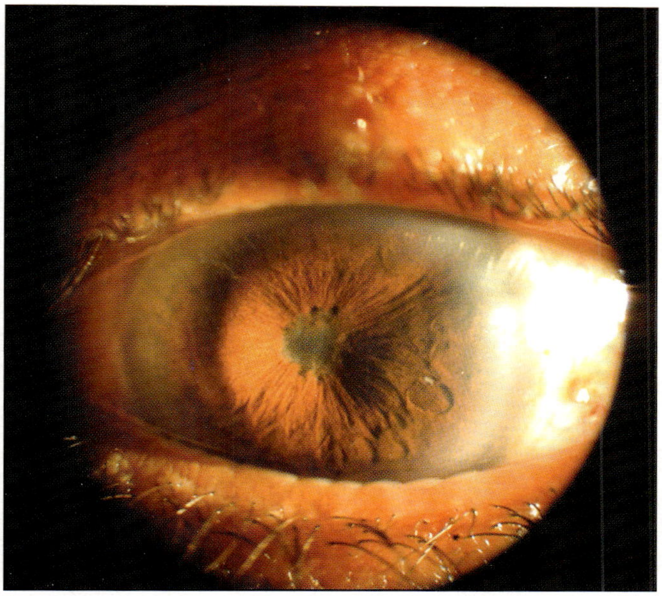

Fig. 25.1: Slit lamp photograph of iris bombe following an attack of acute fibrinous anterior uveitis

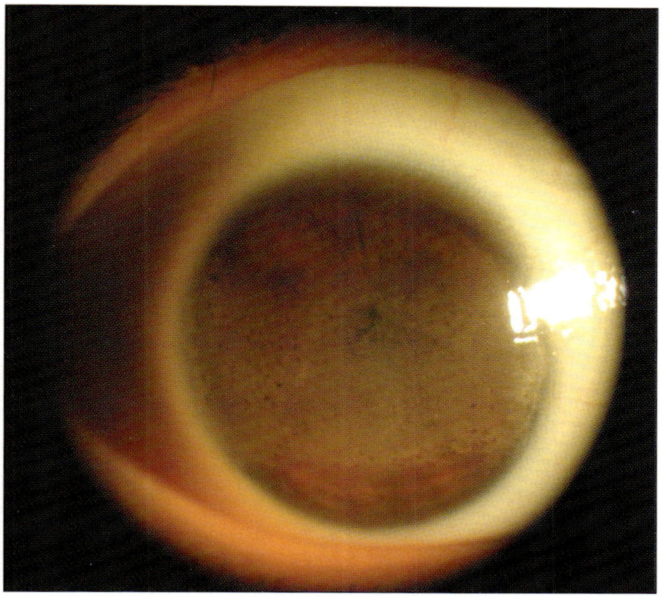

Fig. 25.2: Band keratopathy in a chronic uveitic eye

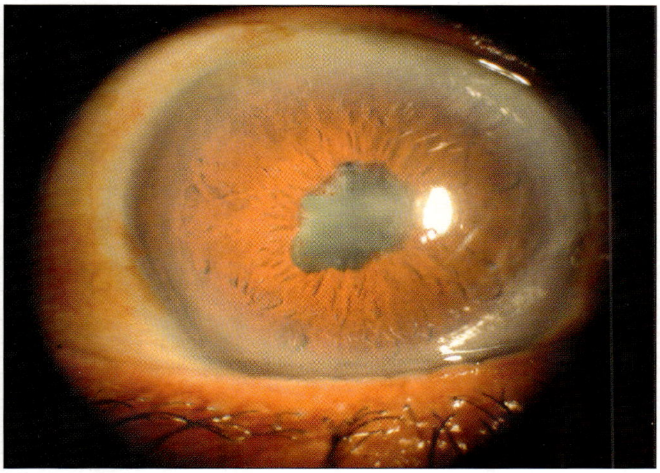

Fig. 25.3: Seclusio pupillae following recurrent attacks of nongranulomatous inflammation

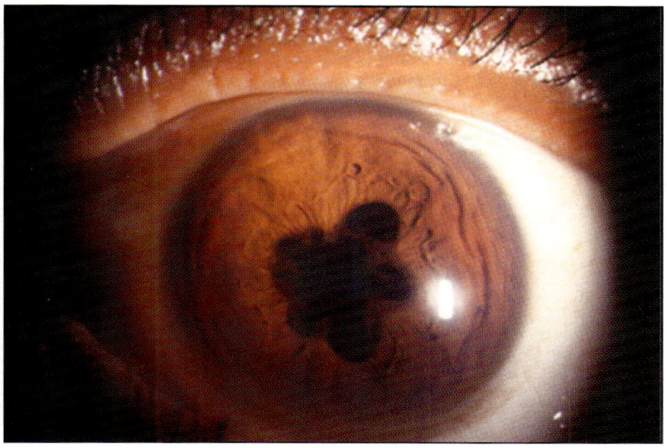

Fig. 25.4: Festooned pupil in chronic anterior uveitis

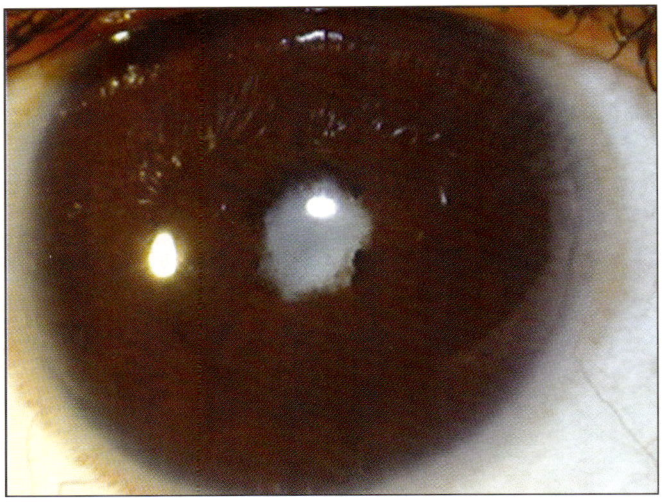

Fig. 25.5: Occlusio pupillae showing a whitish membrane covering the pupillary area

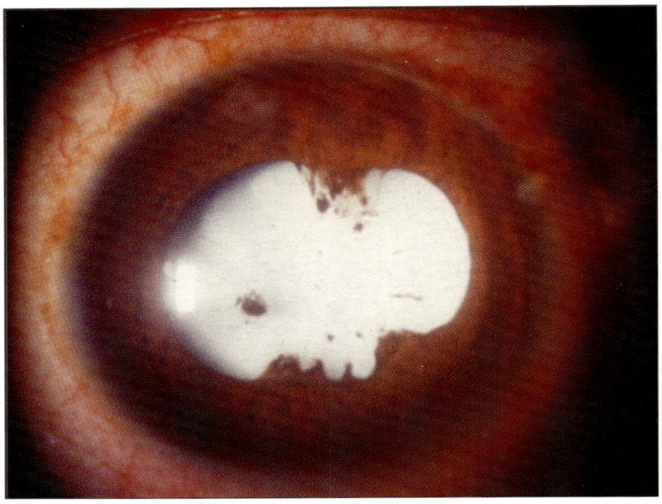

Fig. 25.6: Complicated total cataract with dense posterior synechiae in a young male diagnosed to have HLA B 27 related anterior uveitis

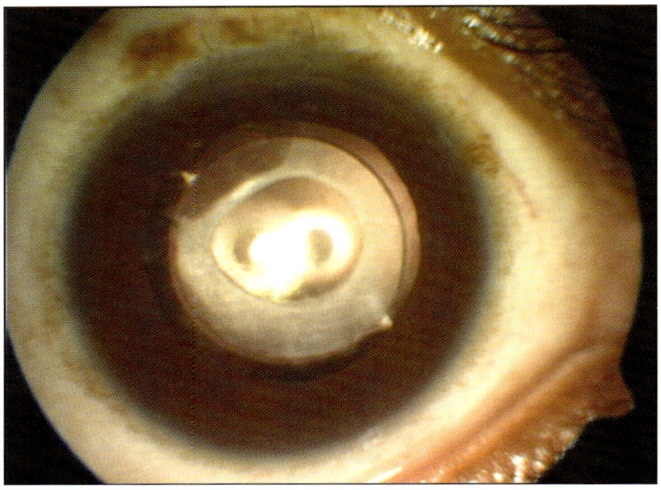

Fig. 25.7: Anterior capsular fibrosis following cataract extraction in a patient with chronic uveitis

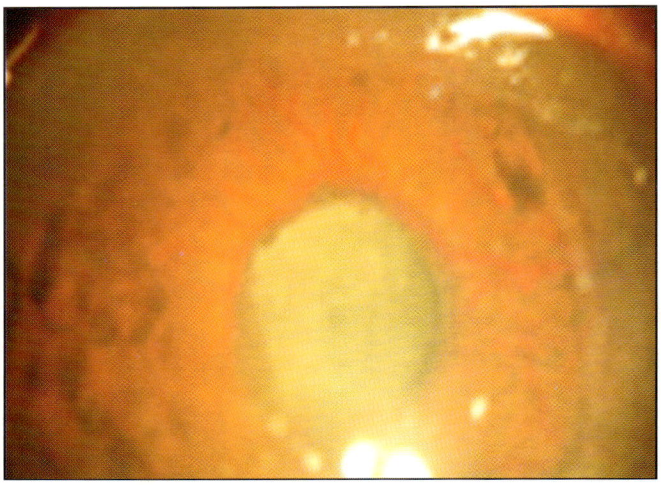

Fig. 25.8: Clinical photograph showing extensive rubeosis iridis with complicated cataract in a patient with severe uveitis

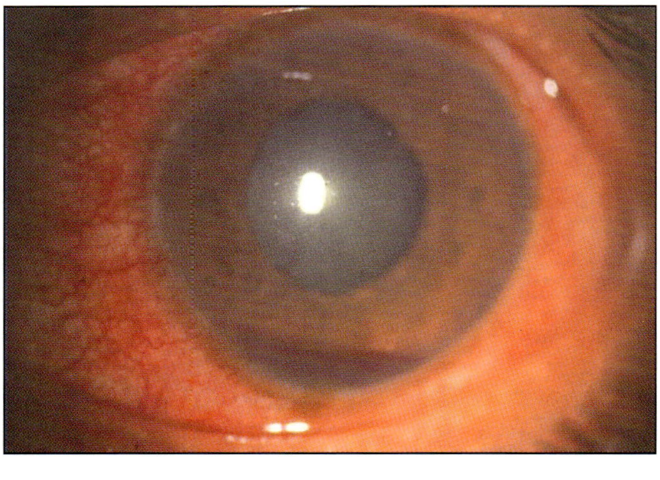

Fig. 25.9: Hyphema in anterior uveitis

Posterior Segment Complications in Uveitis

Choroidal Neovascular Membrane

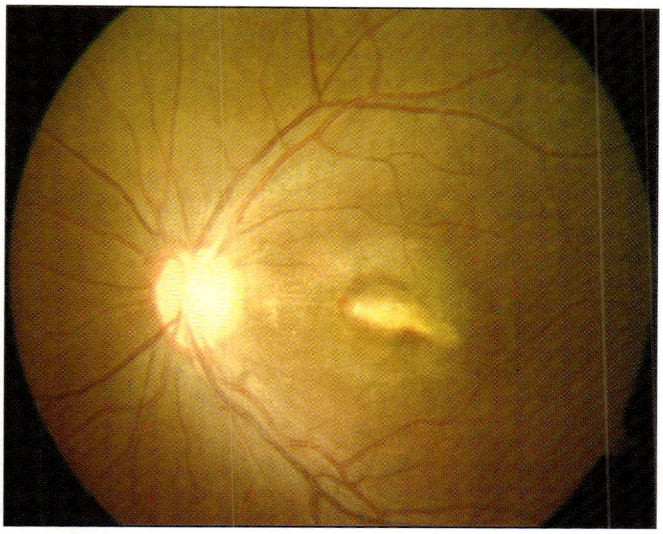

Fig. 25.10: Choroidal neovascular membrane in an eye with resolved choroiditis

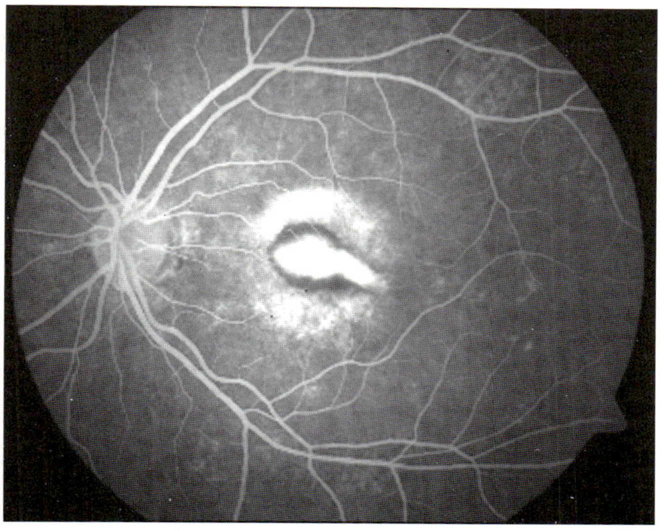

Fig. 25.11: Fluorescein angiogram shows blocked fluorescence due to subretinal hemorrhage and staining of the choroidal neovascular membrane in the late phase

Cystoid Macular Edema

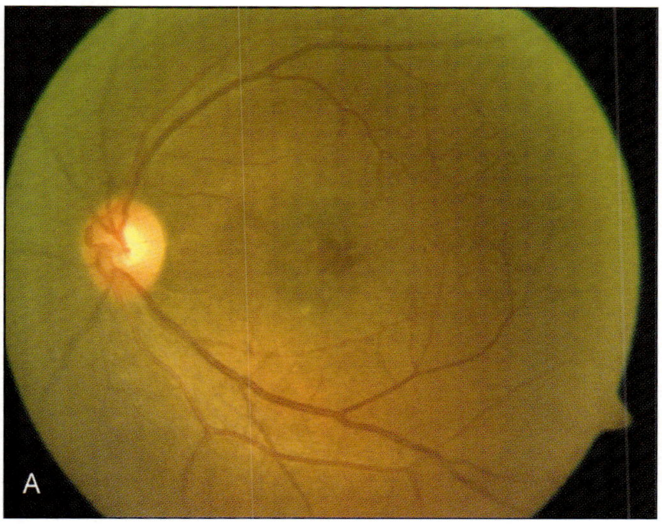

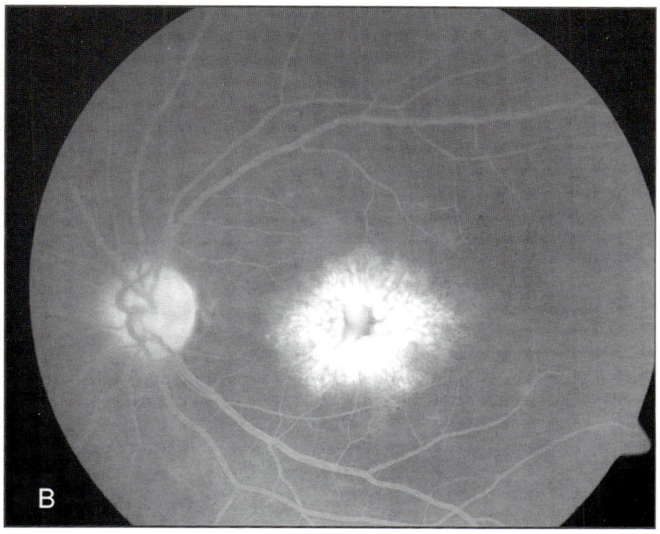

Figs 25.12A and B:

A. Fundus photograph of a 40-year-old patient who developed cystoid macular edema due to chronic intermediate uveitis

B. Fluorescein angiogram showed classical petalloid hyperfluorescence in the late phase

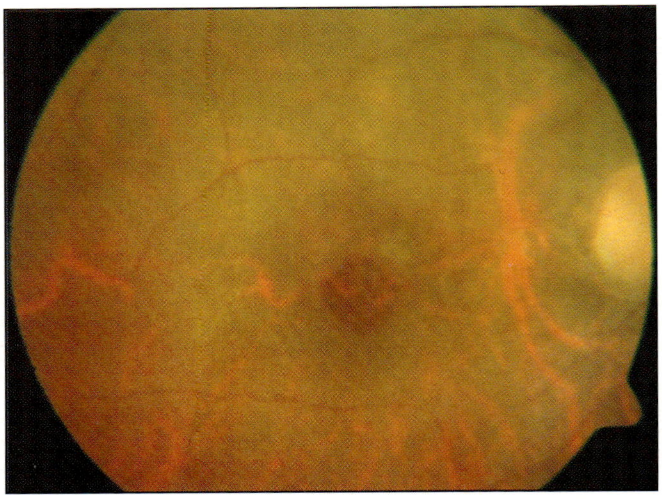

Fig. 25.13: Macular hole and optic atrophy in a patient with Behçet's disease

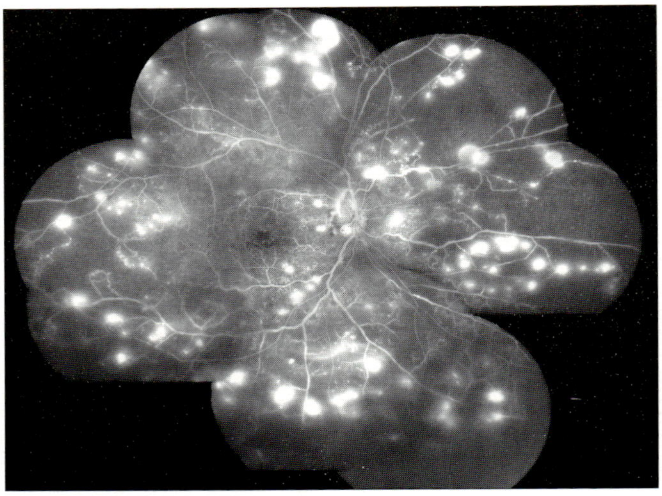

Fig. 25.14: Neovascularization of disc

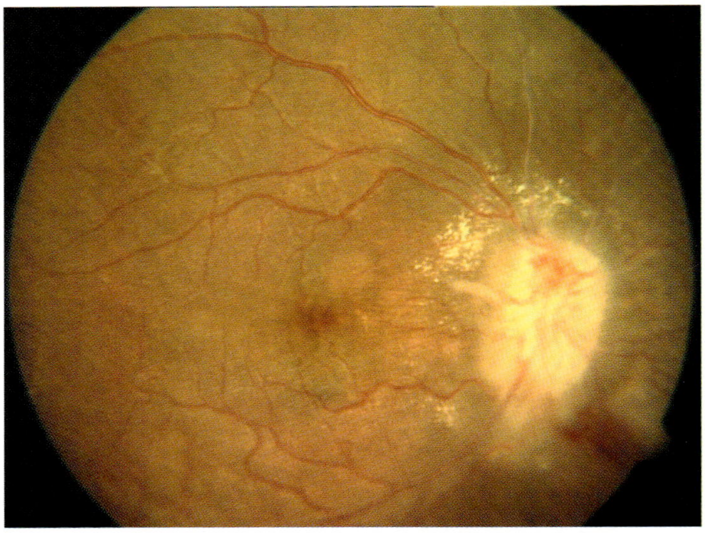

Fig. 25.15: Neovascularization of retina in Eales' disease

Section 8
Investigations in Uveitis

CHAPTER TWENTY SIX

Investigations in Uveitis

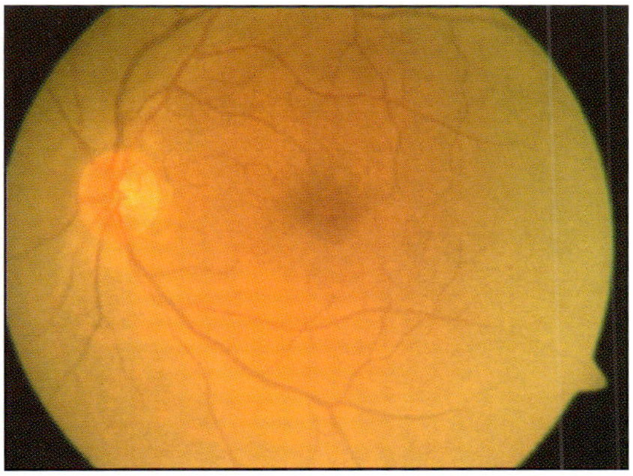

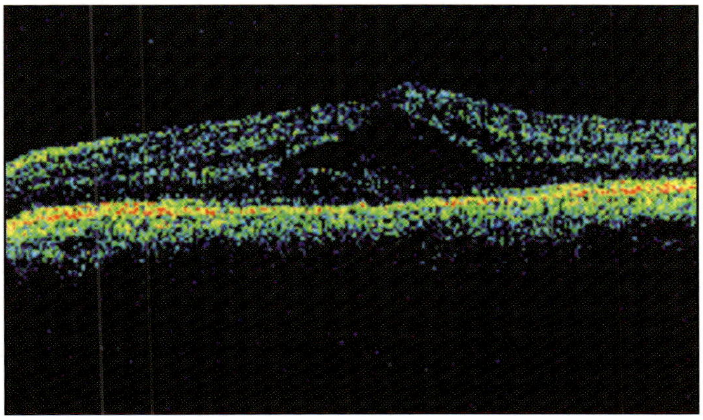

LABORATORY INVESTIGATIONS

Blood Investigations

- Total and differential white blood cell count
- Erythrocyte sedimentation rate

Immunological Tests

- Antinuclear antibodies (ANA)
- Rheumatoid factor (RA)
- Antineutrophilic cytoplasmic antibody
- Human leukocyte antigens (HLA)
  - HLA A 29—Birdshot chorioretinopathy
  - HLA B 27—Ankylosing spondylitis, reiter's syndrome, inflammatory bowel disease, psoriatic arthritis
  - HLA B51—Behcet's syndrome
- Enzyme linked-immunosorbent assay (ELISA) Toxoplasma, toxocara, HIV
- Rapid plasma reagin (RPR)
- Fluorescent treponemal antibody absorption test (FTA Abs)

Biochemical Tests

- Serum angiotensin converting enzyme (ACE)
- Mantoux test
- Polymerase chain reaction

FUNDUS FLUORESCEIN ANGIOGRAPHY (FFA)

Angiography of retinal and choroidal circulation helps in evaluation of posterior segment disorders. FFA is very useful in inflammatory diseases due to its ability to visualize retinal vessels and delineate their walls. The inflammation of retinal vessels alters the endothelial tight junctions due to which fluorescein leaks from the vessels. Thus, vasculitis can be diagnosed well before it is seen clinically. FFA also helps in assessing the leakage of dye from the retinal capillaries in the macula and optic disc in cystoid macular edema and papillitis respectively. Presence of retinal vascular occlusion with retinal and choroidal neovascularization can be easily seen with fluorescein angiography. It is also useful in neurosensory retinal detachment and outer retinal inflammation particularly involving the retinal pigment epithelium. FA is helpful in differentiating active lesion from healed one in retinal and choroidal diseases. In active stage, the margin of the lesion shows diffuse staining and blurring. Healed stage shows hyperfluorescence with well-defined margins. The major drawback of FFA is its inability to image the choroid and detect inflammatory conditions affecting the choroid and choriocapillaris. Also accumulation of blood or pigments prevents the study of any underlying structures by FFA. Posterior uveitic entities in which fluorescein angiography is indicated are:

1. Geographic helicoid peripapillary choroiditis
2. Sarcoidosis
3. Acute posterior multifocal placoid pigment epitheliopathy
4. Multiple evanescent white dot syndrome
5. Sympathetic ophthalmia
6. Vogt-Koyanagi-Harada syndrome
7. Retinal vasculitis
8. Birdshot retinochoroidopathy
9. Behçet's disease
10. Inflammatory CNVM

REFERENCES

1. De Laey JJ. Fluorescein angiography in posterior uveitis. Int Ophthalmol Clin1995;35:33-58.
2. Ben Ezra D. Diagnostic intraocular interventions. In:BenEzra D, Eds. Ocular inflammation:Basic and clinical concepts. Martin Dunitz Ltd 1999: 83-89.

INDOCYANINE GREEN ANGIOGRAPHY (ICGA)

This technique which images the choroid and its associated pathological conditions was introduced in 1970 by Flower and Hochheimer. It uses a tricarbocyanine dye (indocyanine green) which is 98 percent protein bound and operates in infrared range. The dye absorbs light at 790 nm and emits at 830 nm near infrared wavelength. It leaks through the fenestrated choriocapillaries, thus allowing visualization of choroidal circulation through retinal pigment epithelium. ICGA helps in evaluating inflammation and ischemia of large and small choroidal vasculature along with space occupying lesions of choroidal stroma. Choroidal inflammatory lesions are mostly seen as areas of hypofluorescence in indocyanine green angiography. Various inflammatory conditions where ICGA is advised are:

1. Multifocal choroiditis
2. Acute posterior multifocal placoid pigment epitheliopathy
3. Multiple evanescent white dot syndrome
4. Birdshot chorioretinopathy
5. Geographic helicoid peripapillary choroiditis

REFERENCES

1. Herbort CP, LeHoang P, Guex-Crosier Y. Schematic interpretation of indocyanine green angiography in posterior uveitis using a standard angiographic protocol. Ophthalmology 1998;105:432-40.
2. Howe L, Stanford M, Graham E et al. Indocyanine green angiography in inflammatory eye disease. Eye 1998;12:761-67.

B SCAN ULTRASONOGRAPHY

This is a safe, noninvasive and rapid imaging modality which uses frequencies in the range of 7.5-15 MHz for evaluation of posterior globe and orbit. In patients with uveitis, it assesses the inflammatory choroidal and scleral thickening as is seen in posterior scleritis, sympathetic ophthalmia and Vogt-Koyanagi-Harada's disease. Widening of subtenons space also called 'T' sign is especially seen in posterior scleritis. Ultrasound examination also evaluates the posterior segment in conditions with media opacities such as complicated cataract, vitreous hemorrhage, dense vitritis, corneal opacity or miosed pupils.

ULTRASOUND BIOMICROSCOPY (UBM)

It is a relatively new development in the imaging of eye which uses ultrasound frequencies in the range of 50-100 MHz. It allows high resolution examination of anterior 4 mm of the globe, i.e. anterior segment and ciliary body. UBM helps in imaging pars plana exudates in intermediate uveitis particularly if associated with seclusio and occlusio pupillae and complicated cataract obscuring the view of the peripheral fundus. Ciliary body detachment in patients with uveitic hypotony can also be noted on ultrasound biomicroscopy. In cases of IOL induced uveitis, UBM can be used to evaluate the location of the haptic. It has also been used in ciliary body metastatic tumors, which can masquerade as uveitic entities and for diagnosis of pars planitis caused by caterpillar hair or foreign body.

OPTICAL COHERENCE TOMOGRAPHY (OCT)

OCT is a relatively new method of high resolution cross-sectional imaging of the retina. It is based on the principle of low coherence interferometry in near infrared range to achieve high resolution of 10-14 mm. It directly measures the thickness of the retina. It uses the projection of a laser slit beam onto the retina with differential analysis of the reflected light. It is a noninvasive technique. The media should be clear to get retinal image. In uveitis, OCT is particularly useful in the diagnosis and follow-up of cystoid macular edema, macular hole and epiretinal membrane.

REFERENCES

1. Pavin CJ, Harasiewicz K, Sherar MD. Clinical use of ultrasound microscopy. Ophthalmology 1991;98: 287-95
2. Bhende M, Biswas J, Sharma T et al. Ultrasound microscopy in the diagnosis and management of pars planitis caused by caterpillar hairs. Am J Ophthalmol . 2000;125-26.
3. Tran VT, LeHoang P, Herbort CP. Value of high frequency ultrasound microscopy in uveitis. Eye 2001;15 (pt. 1):23-30.

INTRAOCULAR FLUID STUDY

ANTERIOR CHAMBER PARACENTESIS

It is a relatively simple and safe procedure which can be performed by an experienced ophthalmologist. It can be done at the slit lamp or under a microscope in an operation theater after putting antibiotic and anesthetic drops. About 0.1-0.3 ml aqueous fluid is collected with a 27 G needle attached to a tubercular or a 2 cc syringe. The eye is subsequently patched after instillation of antibiotic drops. Aqueous aspirate is then subjected to microbiological and PCR studies.

VITREOUS TAP AND DIAGNOSTIC VITRECTOMY

Vitreous fluid analysis is considered in severe sight threatening uveitis in diagnostic dilemmas and masquerade syndrome where empirical medical treatment has failed to control intraocular inflammation. This procedure is done in an operation theater under a microscope with the help of local anesthesia. Vitreous tap yields a small amount of sample but a three-port diagnostic vitrectomy, provides 0.5-0.7 ml of undiluted vitreous which can be sent for microbiologic, PCR histopathologic or genetic examination.

RETINAL AND CHORIORETINAL BIOPSY

In diagnostic dilemmas where inflammation is localized to sensory retina and retinal pigment epithelium such as toxoplasmic retinochoroiditis, herpes simplex and varicella zoster retinitis, cytomegalovirus retinitis, tubercular or fungal retinitis, tissue biopsy can be performed in order to understand the disease process and make a definite diagnosis. Injury to optic nerve, macula and blood vessels should be particularly avoided. The biopsy site should be at the border of normal retina and active chorioretinal disease.

POLYMERASE CHAIN REACTION

Polymerase chain reaction (PCR) is a new molecular biological technique which is extremely sensitive, specific and rapid in detecting small amounts of DNA from intraocular specimens. It amplifies genomic sequence of an infectious agent over one million times within hours. It is especially useful in endophthalmitis, atypical toxoplasmic retinochoroiditis, viral retinitis and tubercular uveitis. PCR was used in the detection of *Mycobacterium tuberculosis* complex DNA from aqueous sample of suspected tubercular uveitis in a study by Biswas *et al*. In another study, PCR of vitreous humor from 12 cases of Eales' disease and 45 controls of non-Eales' disease showed that 41 percent of vitreous humor was positive for *Mycobacterium tuberculosis* DNA.

REFERENCES

1. Biswas J, Therese L,Madhavan HN: Use of polymerase chain reaction in the detection of Mycobacterium tuberculosis complex DNA from aqueous sample of suspected tubercular uveitis . Uveitis today. Proceedings of the Fourth International Symposium on Uveitis,Yokohama, Japan, 1997;227-30.
2. Therese KL, Anand AR, Madhavan HN: Polymerase chain reaction in the diagnosis of bacterial endophthalmitis. Br J Ophthalmol 1998; 82:1078-82.
3. Biswas J, Therese L,Madhvan HN: Use of polymerase chain reaction in the detection of Mycobacterium tuberculosis complex DNA from vitreous sample of Eales'disease. Br J Ophthalmol 1999;83:994.

IMAGING TECHNIQUES

- **Chest X-ray—**Tuberculosis, sarcoidosis, Wegener's granulomatosis
- **CT scan chest—**Sarcoidosis
- **Gallium scan—**Sarcoidosis
- **MRI scan—**Multiple sclerosis, miliary tuberculosis, CNS lymphoma, Masquerade syndrome and cerebral toxoplasmosis.

FUNDUS FLUORESCEIN ANGIOGRAPHY

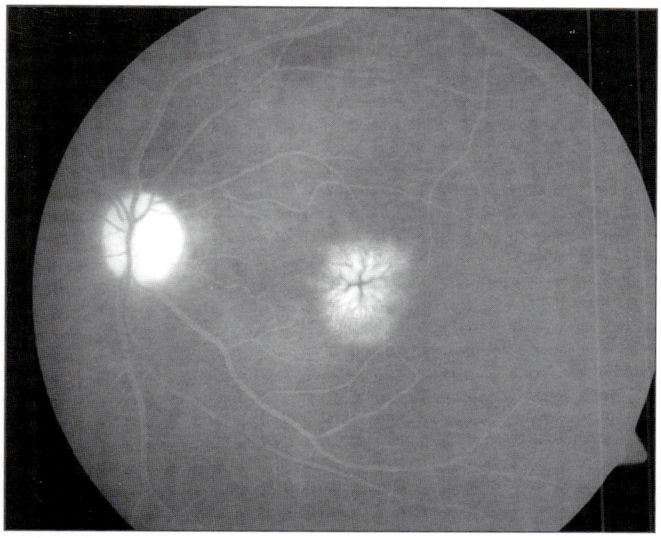

Fig. 26.1: Cystoid macular edema in pars planitis

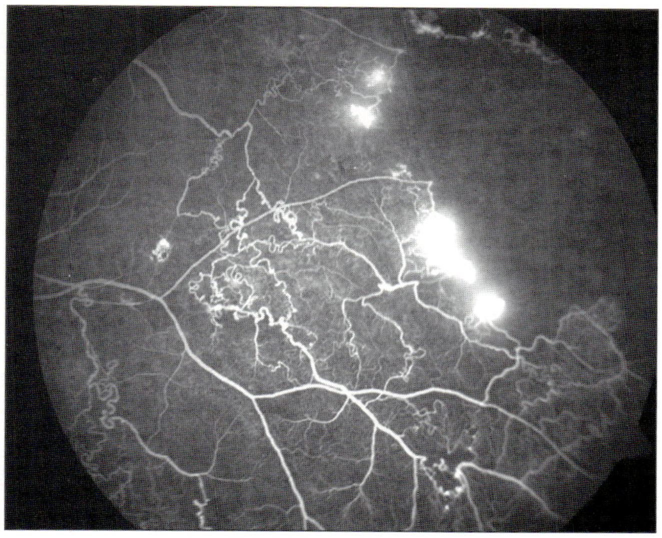

Fig. 26.2: Retinal neovascularization with widespread retinal ischemia in a patient with idiopathic retinal vasculitis

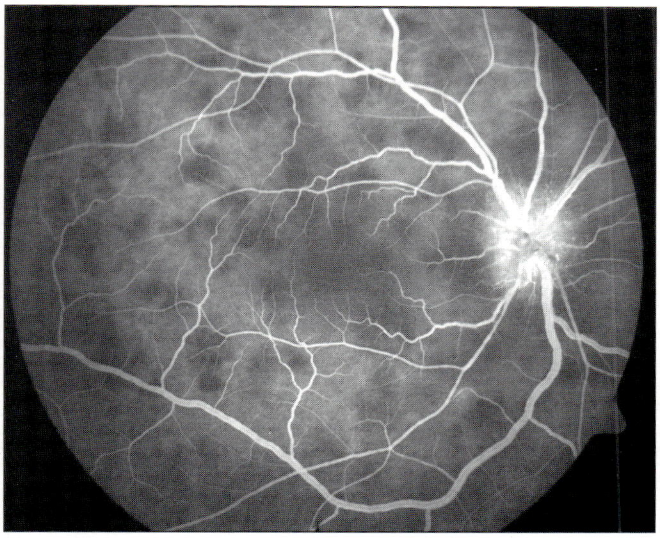

Fig. 26.3: Fluorescein angiogram shows areas of hypofluorescence in arterio venous phase in a patient with multifocal choroiditis

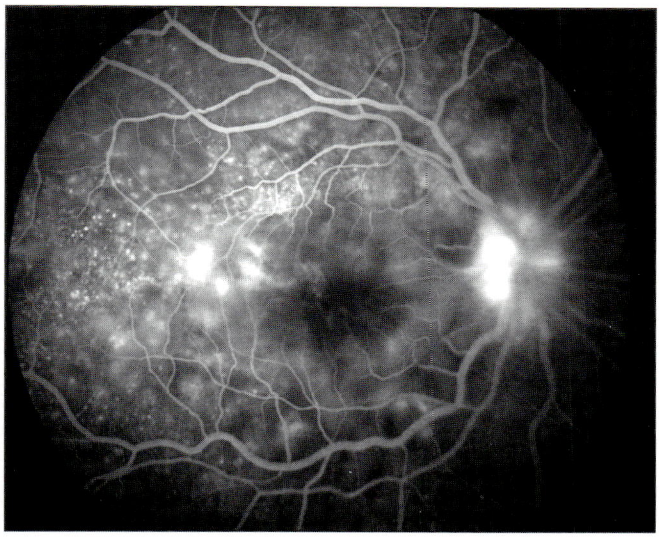

Fig. 26.4: Fluorescein angiogram shows multiple punctate hyperfluorescent dots at the level of RPE with disc leakage in a patient with VKH syndrome

INDOCYANINE GREEN ANGIOGRAPHY

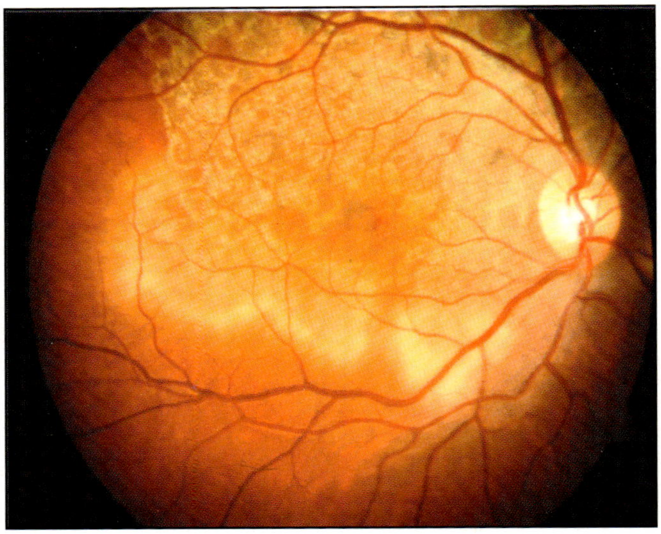

Fig. 26.5: Active serpiginous choroiditis involving the macula

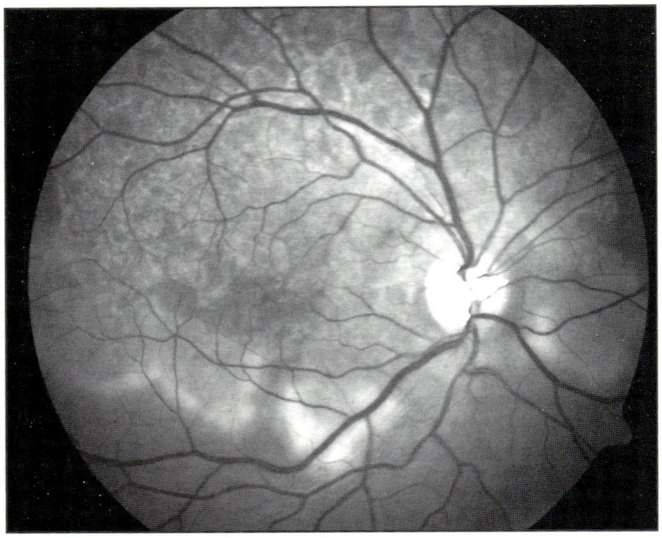

Fig. 26.6: Red free photograph of the same patient

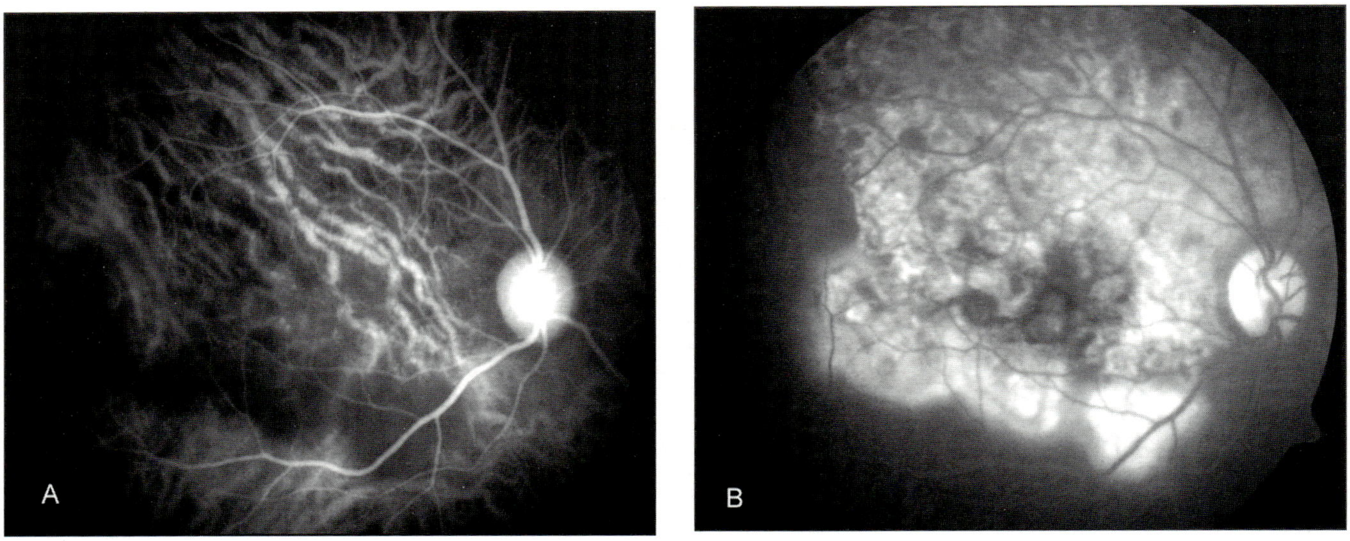

Figs 26.7A and B: ICG angiogram showing early hypofluorescence (A) followed by late staining (B) in active serpiginous choroiditis

B scan Ultrasound

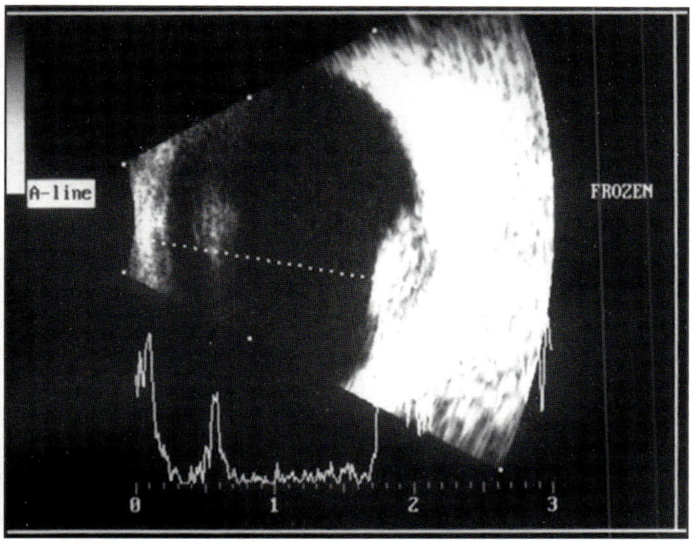

Fig. 26.8: Ultrasound B-scan showing a subretinal mass with high internal reflectivity diagnosed as tubercular abscess

Ultrasound Biomicroscopy

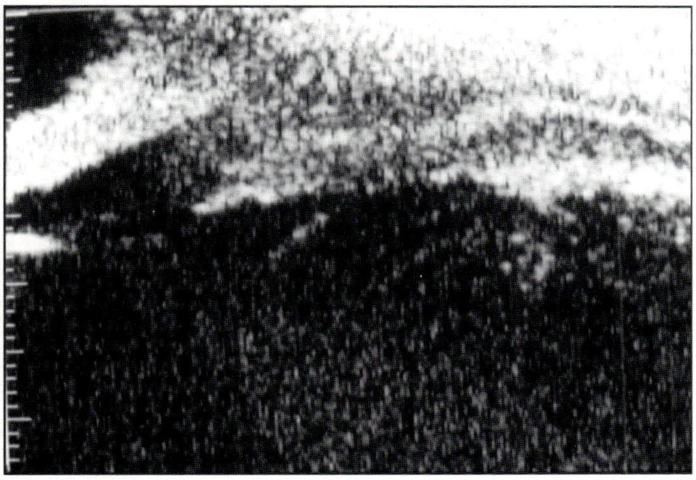

Fig. 26.9: Ultrasound biomicroscopy showing *pars plana* exudates in a case of intermediate uveitis

Optical Coherence Tomography

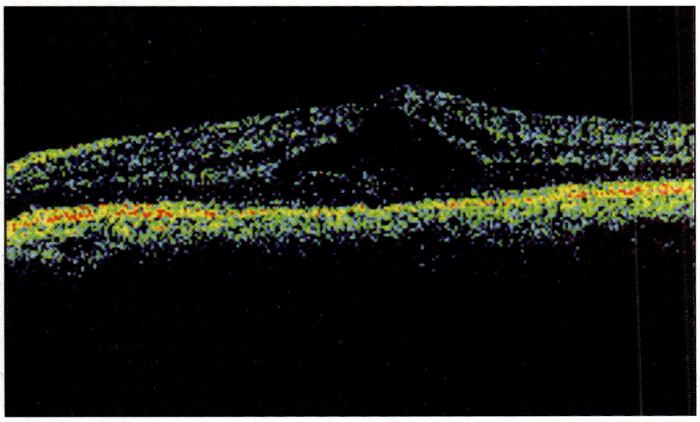

Fig. 26.10: OCT showing cystoid macular edema in a patient with chronic postoperative uveitis

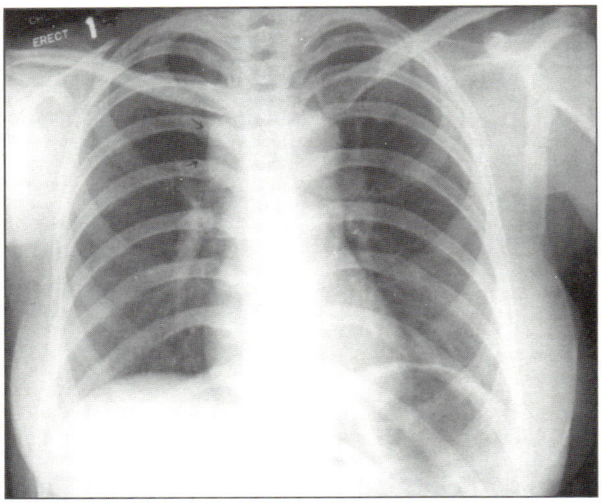

Fig. 26.11: Chest X-ray in a patient with pulmonary tuberculosis

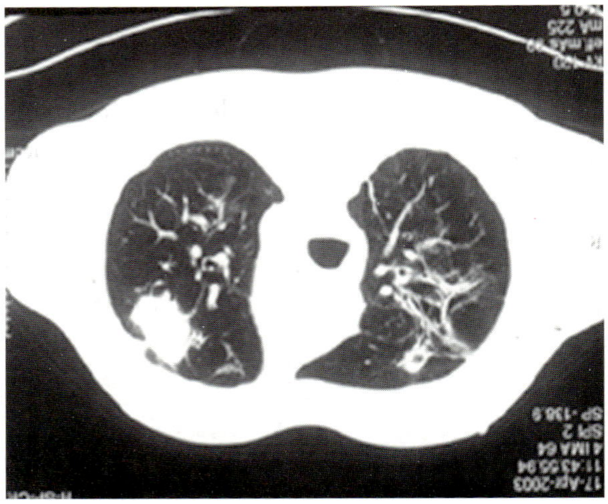

Fig. 26.12: CT scan of chest in a patient with sarcoidosis

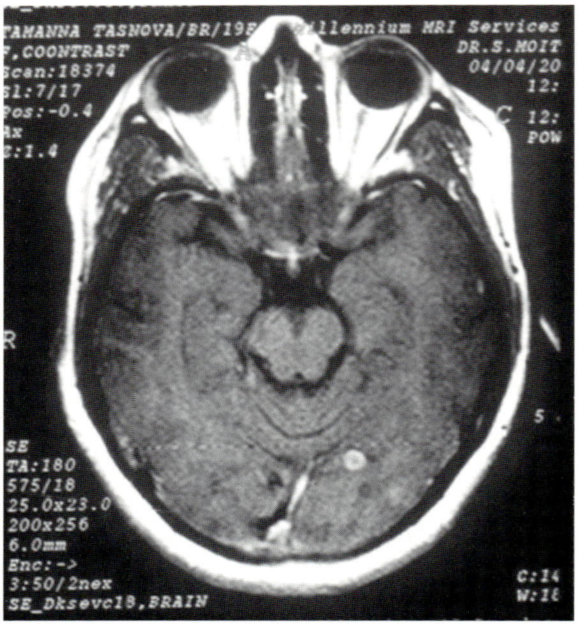

Fig. 26.13: MRI brain in a patient with miliary tuberculosis

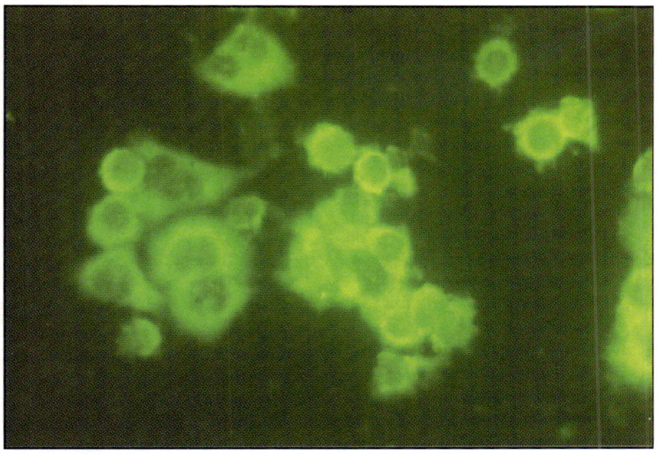

Fig. 26.14: Rim staining of antinuclear antibodies

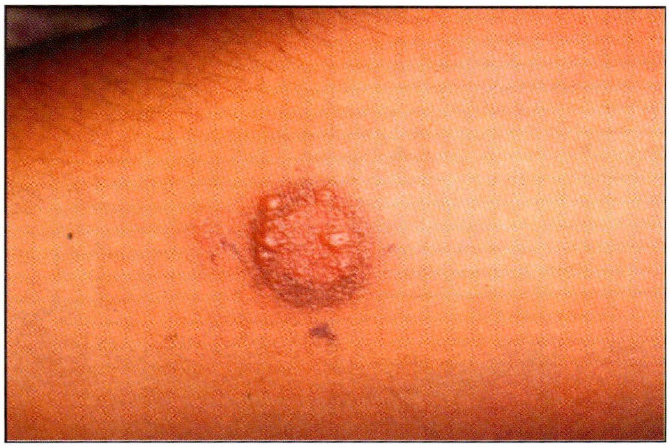

Fig. 26.15: Mantoux test in a patient with tuberculosis showing erythema, induration and bleb formation

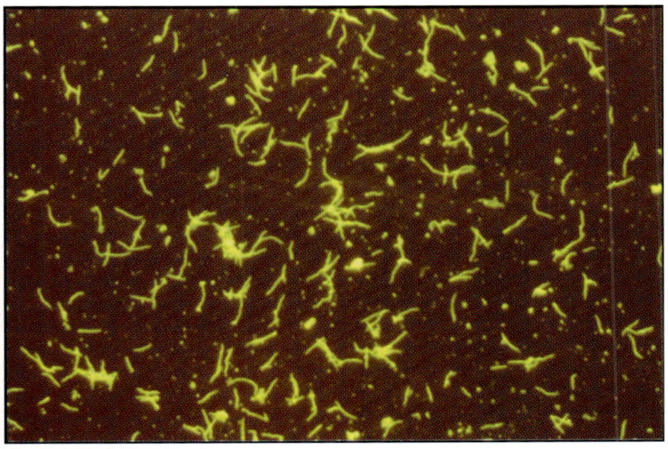

Fig. 26.16: Dark field microscopy showing *Treponema pallidum* in a patient with syphilis

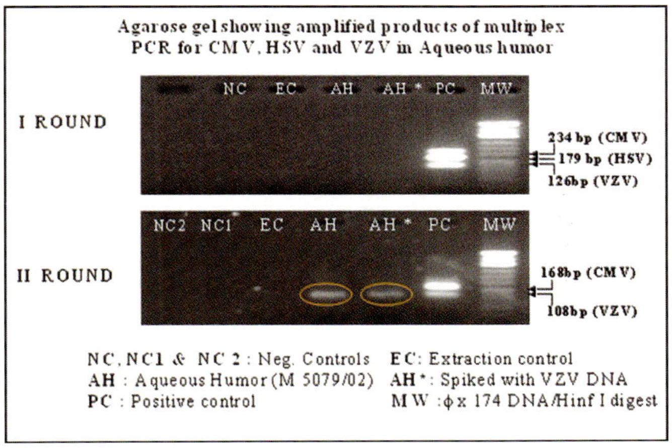

Fig. 26.17: Polymerase chain reaction positive for VZV genome in aqueous aspirate in a patient with acute retinal necrosis

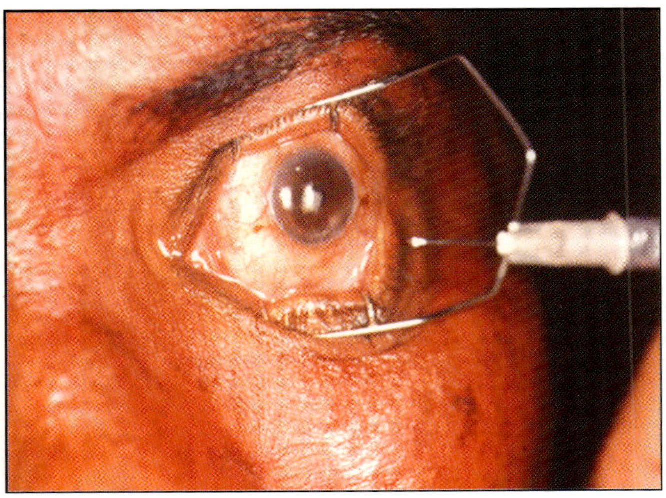

Fig. 26.18: Aqueous tap

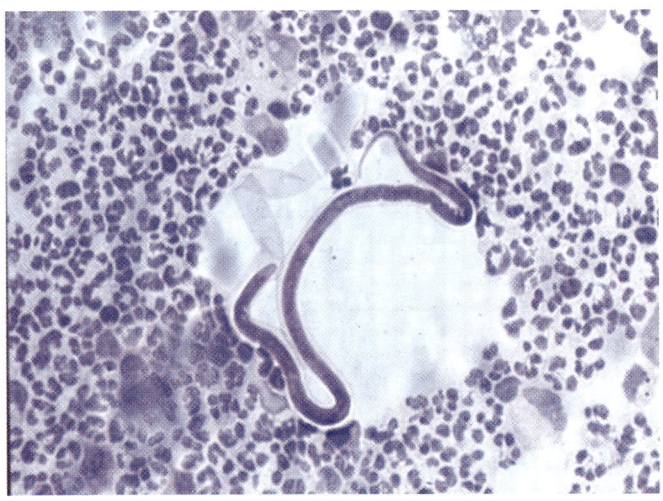

CHAPTER TWENTY SEVEN

Masquerade Syndrome

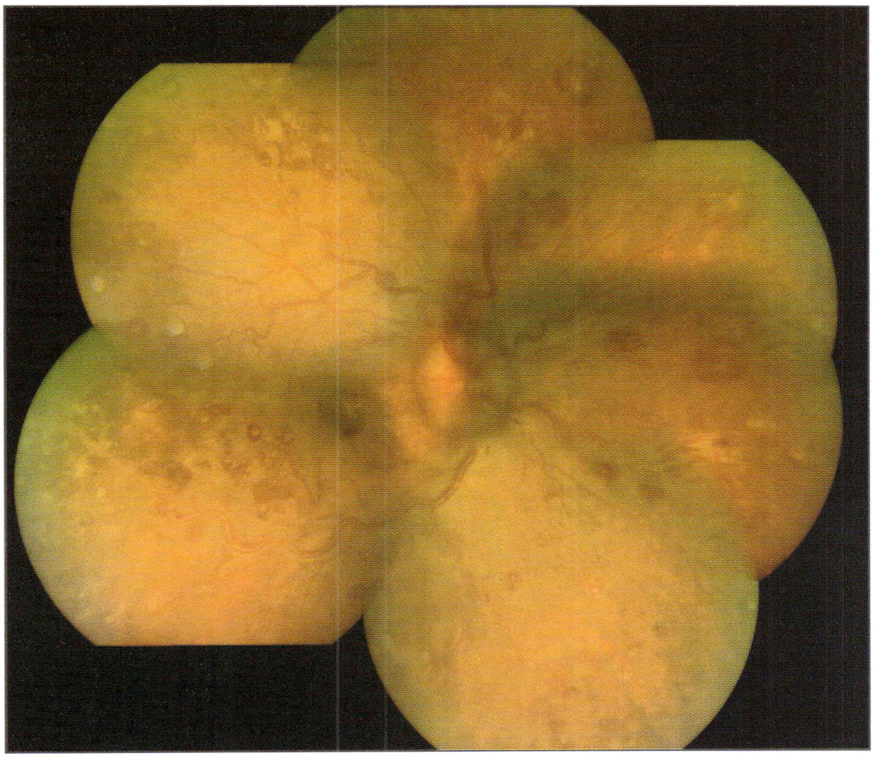

Masquerade syndromes are benign or malignant ocular lesions that mimic intraocular inflammation. It is often suspected when uveitis occurs in very young patients or patients over the age of 60 years. Various syndromes that masquerade as uveitis are:

1. Intraocular lymphoma
2. Retinoblastoma
3. Leukemia
4. Intraocular foreign body
5. Uveal melanoma
6. Juvenile xanthogranuloma
7. Retinitis pigmentosa
8. Retinal detachment

Primary Intraocular Lymphoma

It arises from the eye, brain, spinal cord or leptomeninges. It is usually bilateral and seen in patients over 50 years. Ocular manifestations are seen prior to systemic involvement in 50% -80% cases.

Symptoms: Blurred vision, floaters

Signs: Aqueous cells and flare, large clumps of vitreous cells, multiple large yellowish subretinal and choroidal lesions which are non-responsive to corticosteroids

Investigations

- Diagnostic vitrectomy showing malignant cells
- CT or MRI brain

Treatment

Ocular and CNS irradiation along with intrathecal chemotherapy.

Retinoblastoma

It is the most common primary intraocular malignancy in children and may masquerade as intraocular inflammation in a child less than 5 years.

Symptoms: Leukocoria, strabismus, red eye, decreased vision.

Signs:

- Aqueous cells, flare, pseudohypopyon
- Serous retinal detachment

Investigations

- Ultrasound or CT scan showing intraocular calcification

Treatment

External beam radiation, enucleation, photocoagulation, cryotherapy.

Leukemia

Ocular involvement in leukemias occur either because of infiltration by leukemic cells or due to hemorrhagic phenomenon. It can involve either anterior or posterior segment.

Anterior: Conjunctival injection, iridocyclitis, pseudohypopyon, spontaneous hyphema, heterochromia iridis, glaucoma.

Posterior:

- Vitreous exudates and hemorrhage
- Leukemic retinopathy characterized by tortuous dilated vessels, retinal hemorrhages, roths' spots, and cotton wool spots.
- Optic nerve infiltration and papilloedema may also be seen.

Intraocular foreign body can present as anterior or posterior uveitis.

Juvenile xanthogranuloma usually presents as anterior chamber cells, flare and spontaneous hyphema in a child less than 1 year of age.

Rhegmatogenous retinal detachment results in vitreous reaction presenting as tobacco dust.

REFERENCE

1. Tsai T, O'Brien JM. Masquerade syndromes: malignancies mimicking inflammation in the eye. Int Ophthalmol Clin 2002 ;42:115-31.

A 57-year-old woman presented with blurred vision in both eyes for 8 months. Best corrected visual acuity was hand movements close to face.

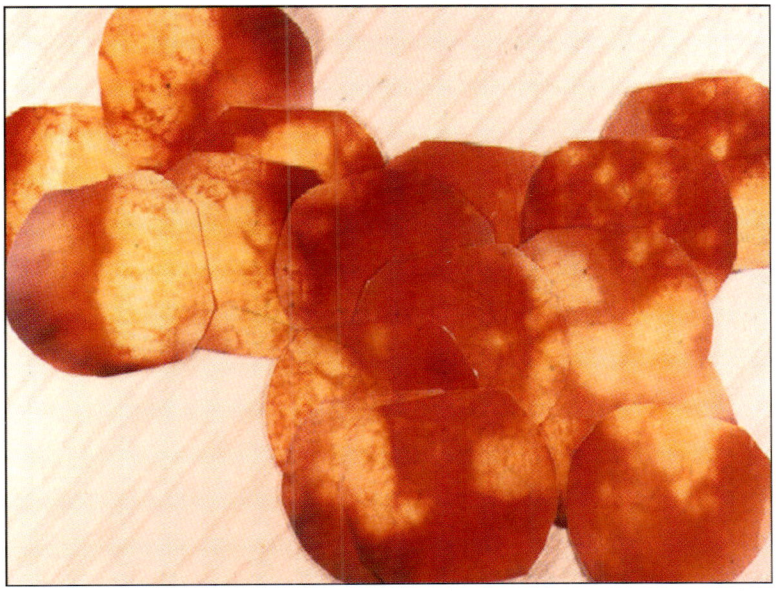

Fig. 27.1: Fundus photograph shows multiple cream colored subretinal lesions scattered throughout the retina

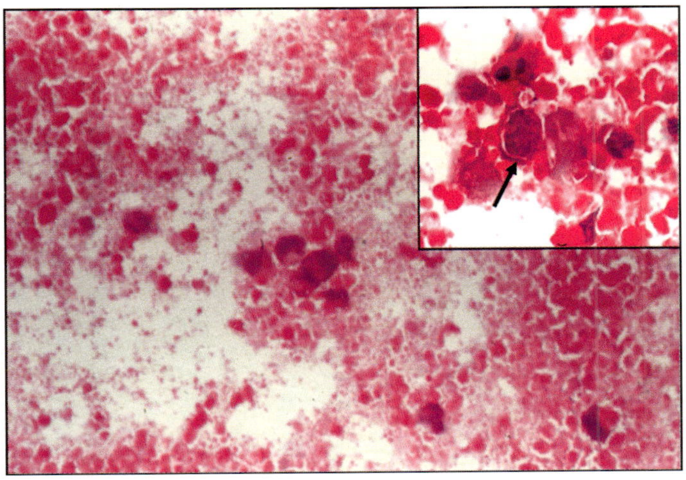

Fig. 27.2: Histopathology of fine needle aspiration biopsy showed necrotic tumor cells, RBCs and malignant large cells with hyperchromatic nuclei and scanty cytoplasm suggestive of large cell lymphoma

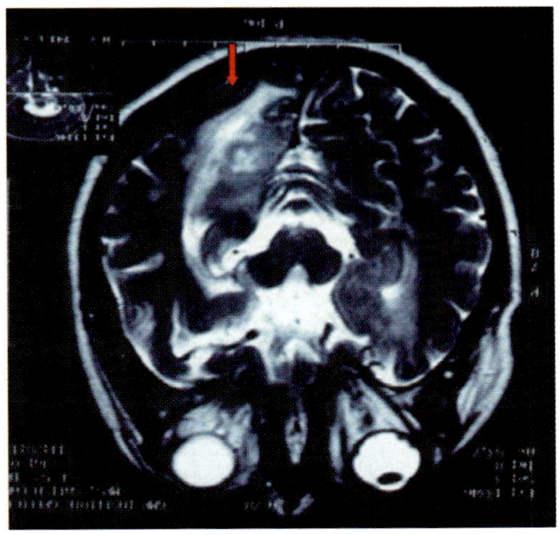

Fig. 27.3: MRI showed multiple lesions in frontal, temporal, occipital, thalamic and periventricular areas of brain

Retinoblastoma

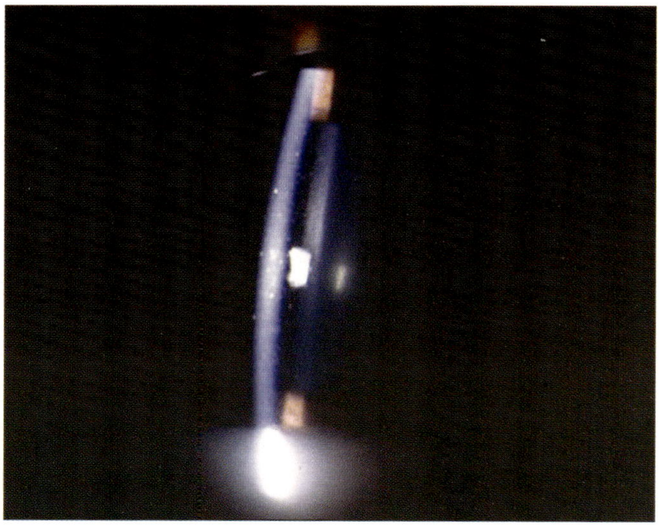

Fig. 27.4: Slit lamp photograph showing hypopyon in a 8-year-old girl

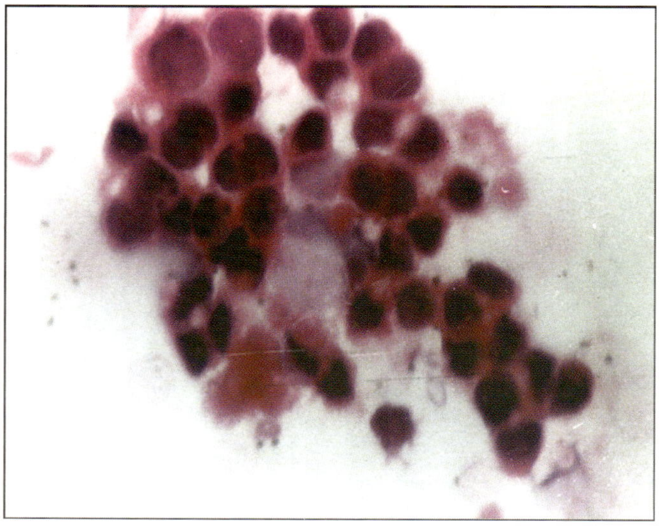

Fig. 27.5: Photomicrograph of aqueous aspirate showing highly cohesive basophilic pleomorphic tumor cells with hyperchromatic nuclei and scanty cytoplasm suggestive of retinoblastoma

Chronic Myeloid Leukemia

A 40-year-old patient came with complaints of mild blurring of vision in both eyes. He also gave a history of weight loss, frequent bruising on trivial injuries and fatigue. Anterior segment examination was normal

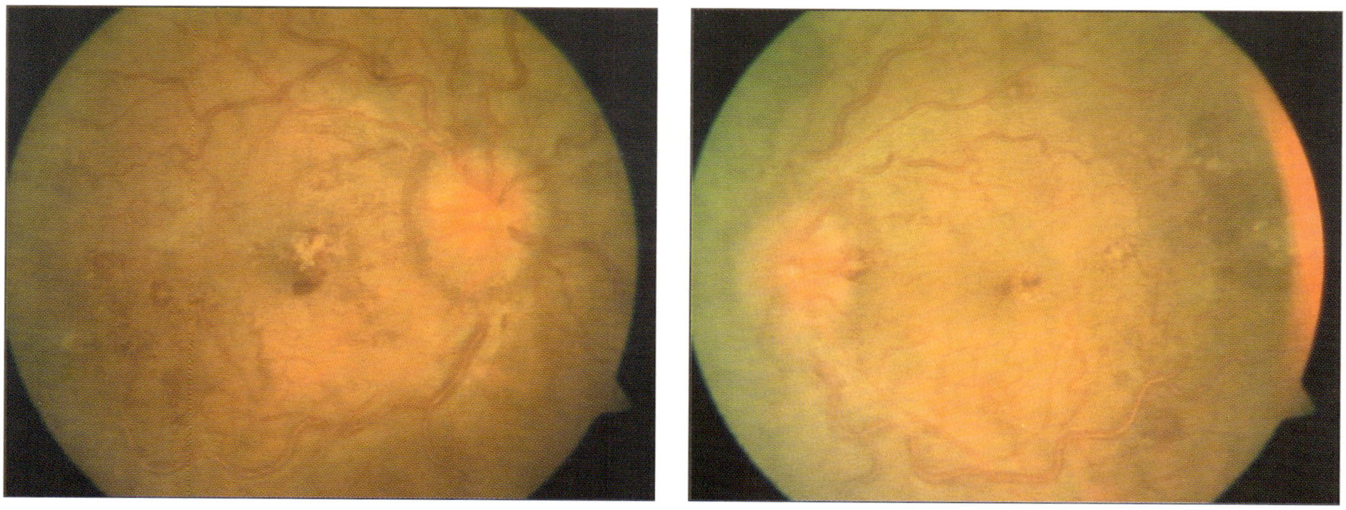

Figs 27.6A and B: Fundus photograph shows bilateral disc edema, dilated tortuous retinal vessels, retinal hemorrhages and Roth's spots. Routine blood investigations showed total white blood cell count 2,40,000 and Hb—8.2%. Peripheral blood smear showed hypochromic microcytic red blood cells and leucocytes with promyelocytes, myelocytes, metamyelocytes and few blast cells suggestive of chronic myeloid leukemia

Section 10
Acquired Immunodeficiency Syndrome (AIDS)

CHAPTER TWENTY EIGHT

Acquired Immunodeficiency Syndrome (AIDS)

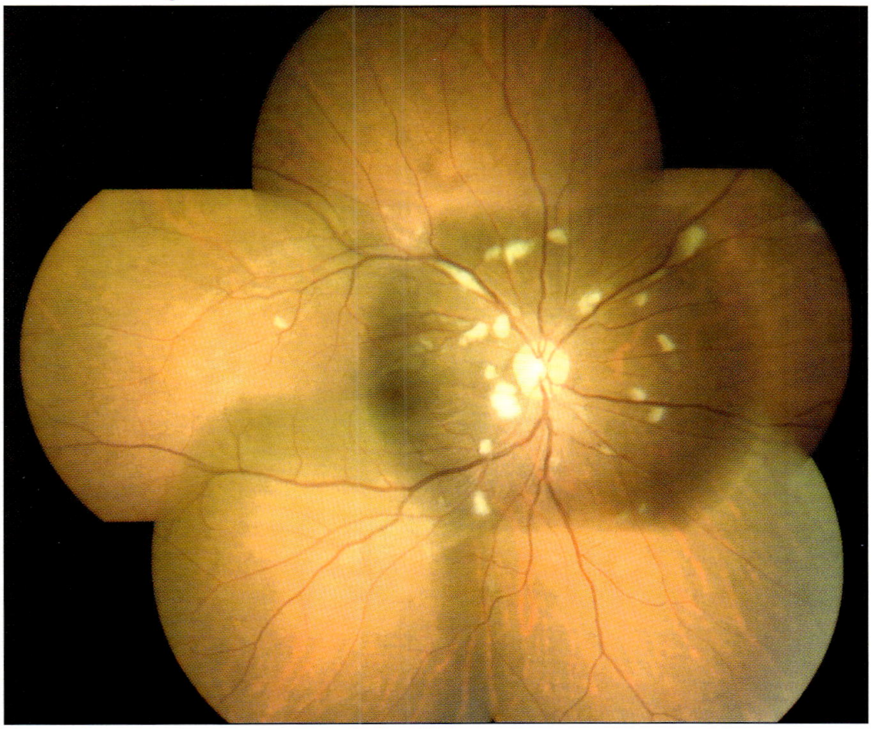

Cytomegalovirus Retinitis in AIDS

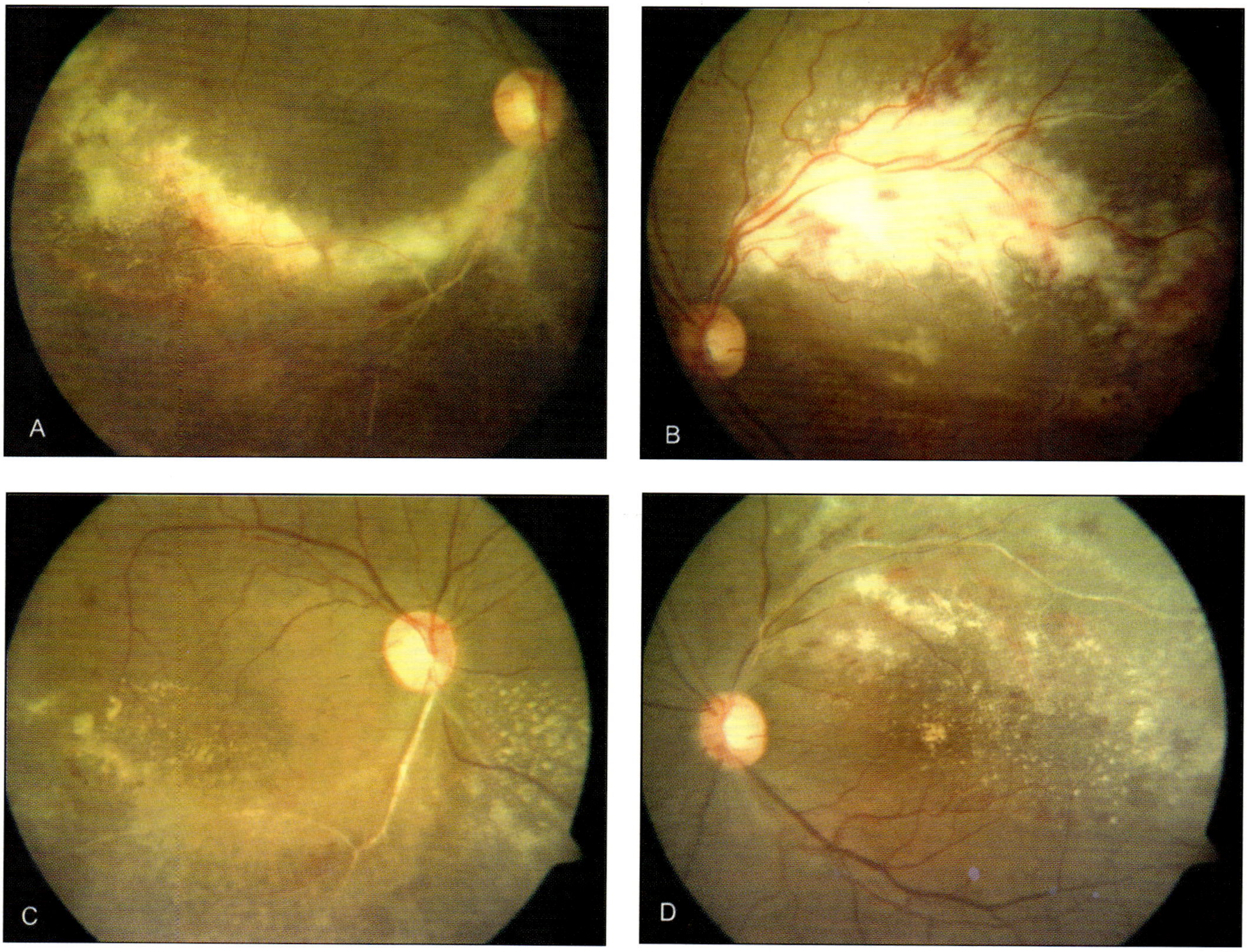

Figs 28.6A to D: A 28-year-old HIV patient, complained of gradual decrease in vision in both eyes for 1 month. His CD4 counts were 83 cells/mm^3. (A and B) Fundus photograph shows areas of retinal necrosis associated with intraretinal hemorrhages and perivasculitis in both the eyes due to cytomegalovirus retinitis. (C and D) Fundus photograph shows marked resolution of the lesions following two weeks of intravenous ganciclovir injections

Frosted Branch Angiitis in AIDS

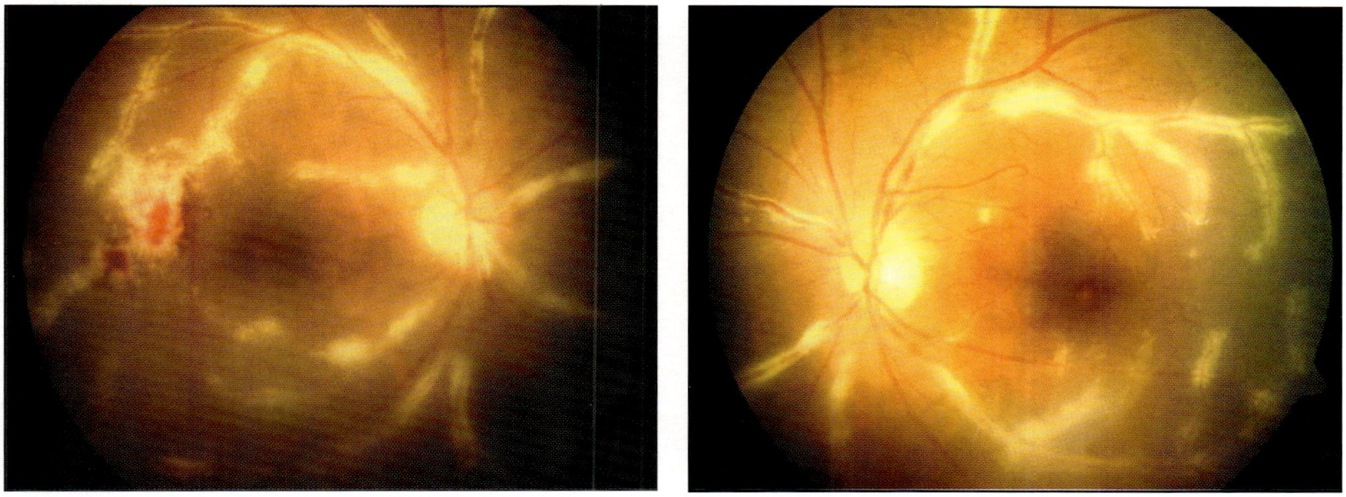

Figs 28.7A and B: Frosted branch angiitis in the right and left eye in an HIV patient with CD 4 counts 50/mm^3

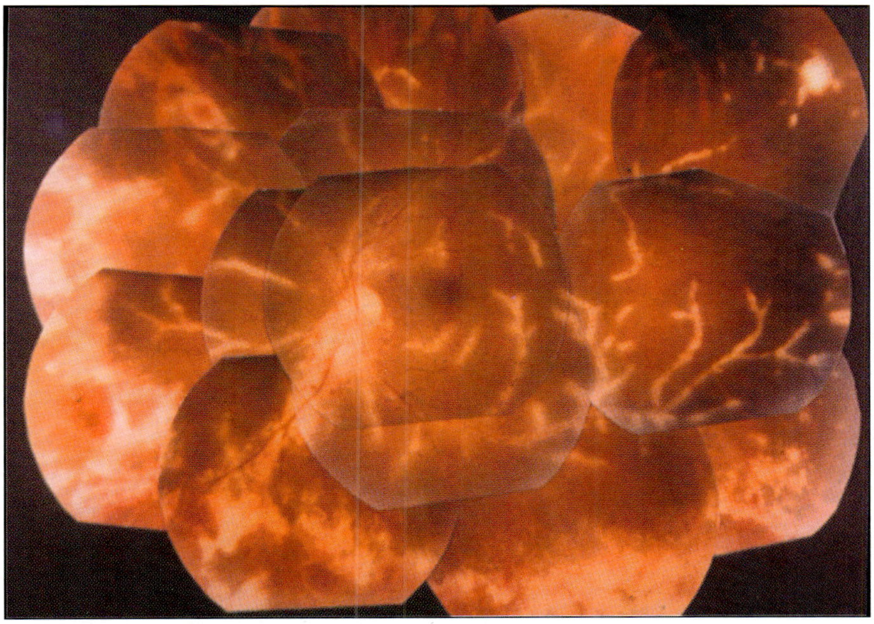

Fig. 28.7C: Montage fundus photograph showing frosted branch angiitis with areas of retinitis in the periphery in an AIDS patient

Progressive Ocular Retinal Necrosis in AIDS

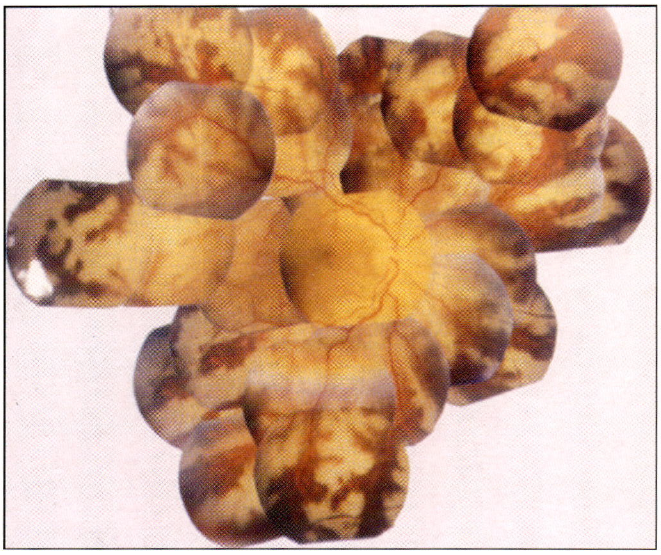

Fig. 28.8: Progressive outer retinal necrosis in an AIDS patient. Note the sparing of the retinal vessels

Acute Retinal Necrosis in AIDS

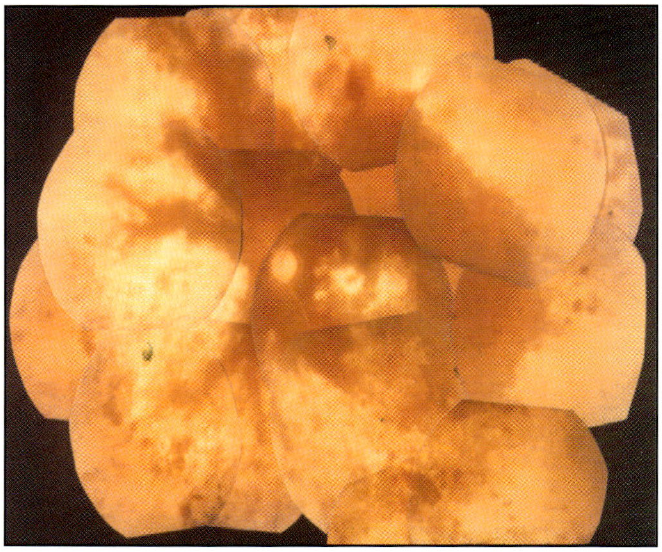

Fig. 28.9: Fundus photograph showing yellowish white peripheral lesions in acute retinal necrosis in an AIDS patient

Toxoplasmic Retinochoroiditis in AIDS

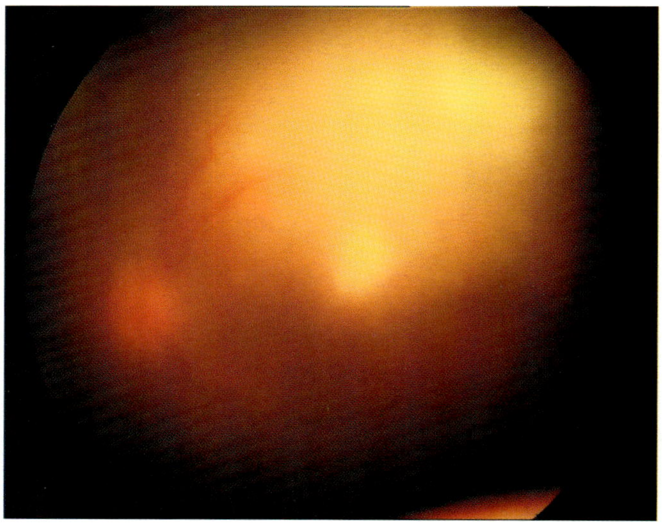

Fig. 28.10: Fundus photograph shows active retinochoroiditis with vitreitis in an HIV+ patient

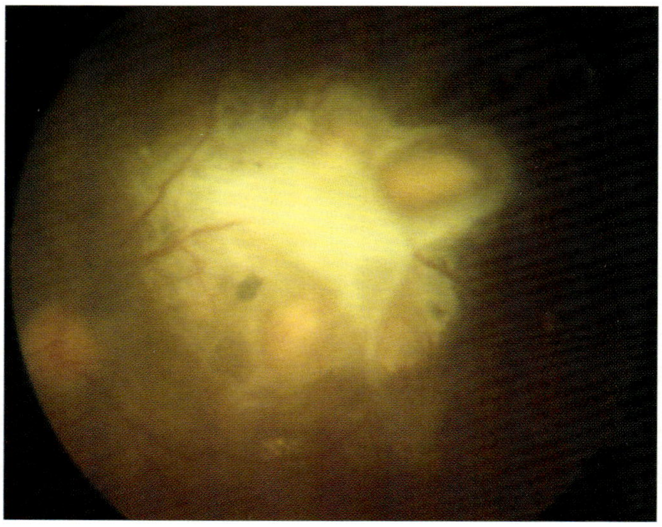

Fig. 28.11: Healed retinochoroiditis scar with gliosis after anti-toxoplasma treatment in the same patient

Ocular Tuberculosis in AIDS

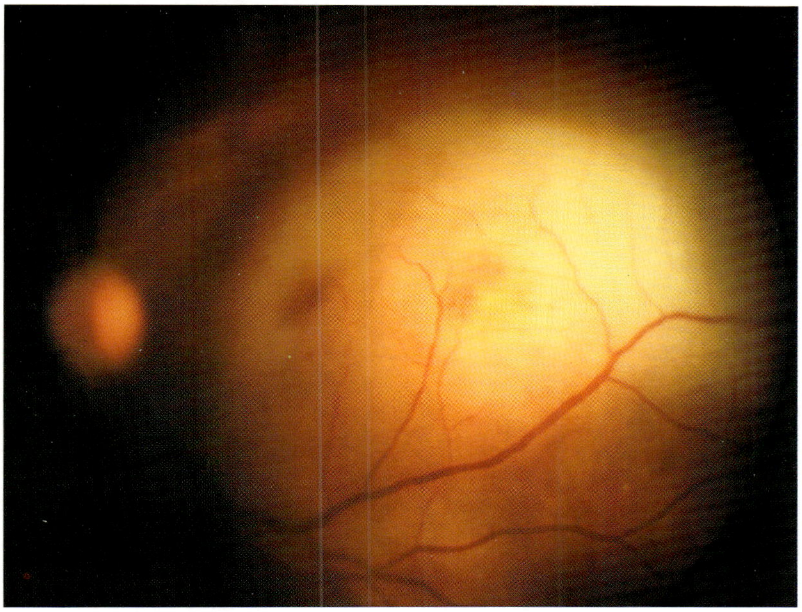

Fig. 28.12: A 34-year-old known HIV patient complained of sudden decrease in vision in left eye for 10 days. Fundus photograph shows a large yellowish sub-retinal abscess in the posterior pole. Fine needle aspiration biopsy showed multiple acid fast bacilli, suggestive of *Mycobacterium tuberculosis*

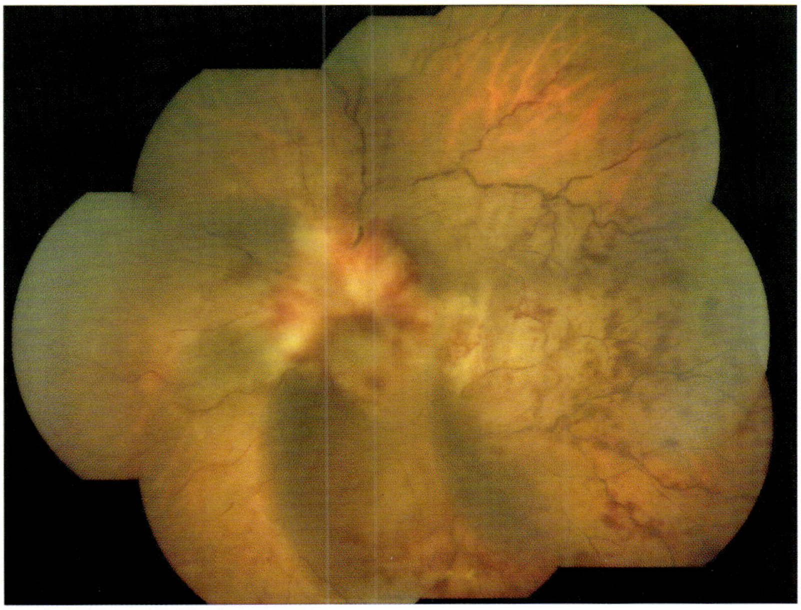

Fig. 28.13: Fundus photograph of a 33-year-old, HIV patient showing disc edema with surrounding flame shaped hemorrhages. The peripheral retina shows scattered hemorrhages with few cuffs of active vasculitis in the inferior quadrant.
MRI of the brain and orbit revealed nodular and ring enhancing lesions in right temporal and left parietal lobe. Also the left optic nerve was found to be thickened. Cerebrospinal fluid tap was done and polymerase chain reaction for *Mycobacterium tuberculosis* was positive.

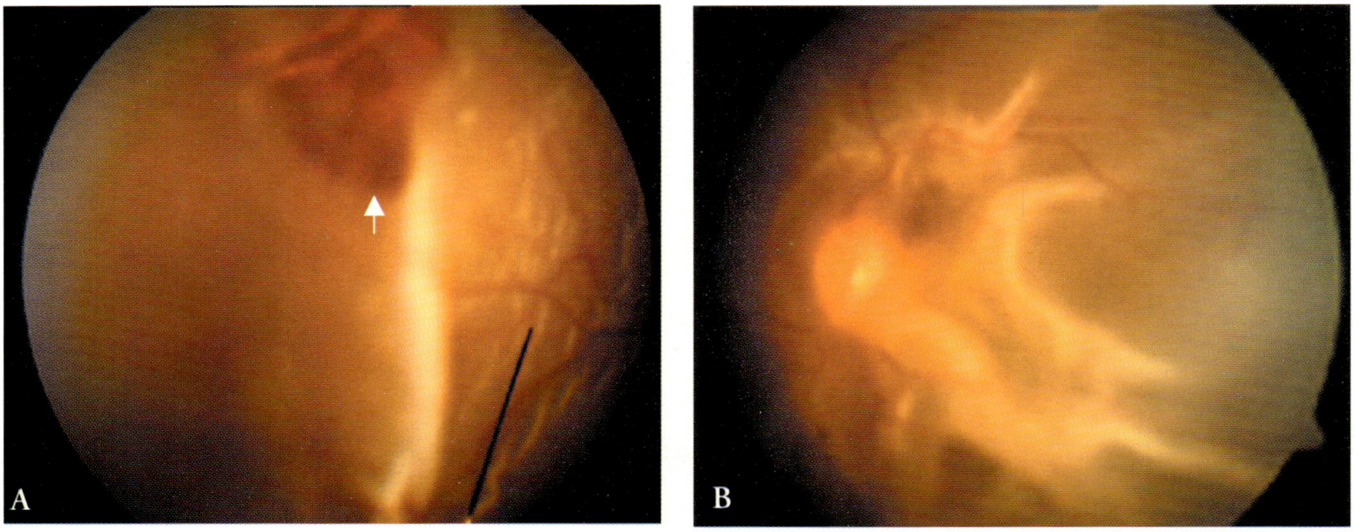

Figs 28.14A and B: A 38-year-old HIV+ patient, complained of sudden diminution of vision in right eye for last 10 days. On examination, his vision in right eye was 6/36 and in left eye was just light perception. (A) Fundus examination in right eye revealed rhegmatogenous retinal detachment with large breaks (arrow) (B) Left eye showed total retinal detachment with multiple breaks due to acute retinal necrosis

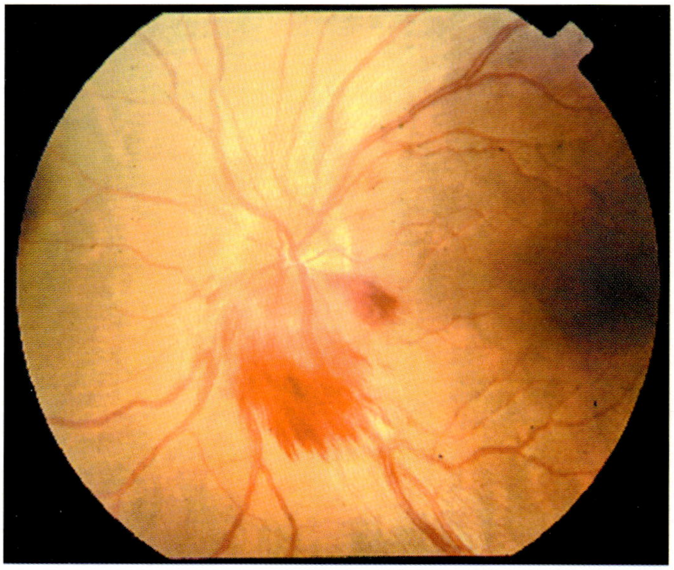

Fig. 28.15: Papilledema with peripapillary hemorrhages in cryptococcal meningitis in an AIDS patient.

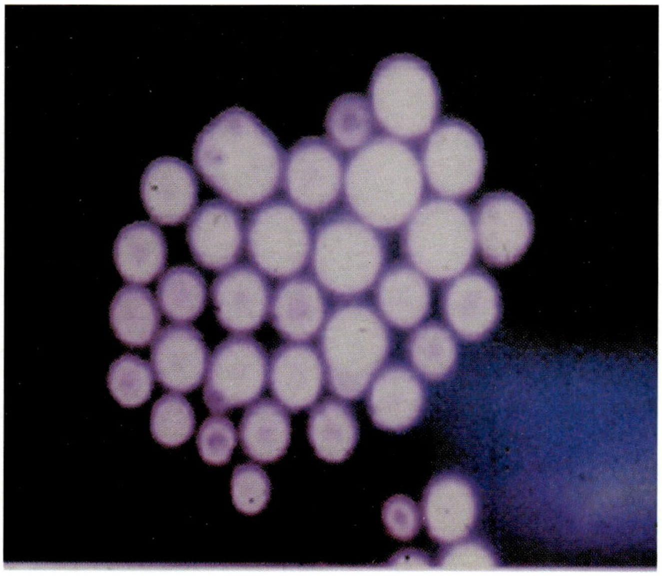

Fig. 28.16: CSF analysis of the same patient showed cryptococcal organism in India ink preparation

Section 11
Scleritis

Scleritis is an inflammatory condition of the eye characterized by edema and inflammatory cell infiltration of the sclera. It is common in the fifth to sixth decades of life and women are more commonly affected than men. Scleritis is frequently associated with systemic diseases in 50 percent cases.

Classification

1. **Anterior scleritis**
   - Diffuse
   - Nodular
   - Necrotizing
     - With inflammation
     - Without inflammation *(Scleromalacia perforans)*
     - Surgically induced necrotizing scleritis
2. **Posterior scleritis**

ANTERIOR SCLERITIS

- **Diffuse anterior scleritis:** A painful, intense inflammation involving both sclera and episclera. A superficial redness may be cleared by vasoconstriction to observe the scleral swelling which is best detected using the slit lamp beam with red free light.
- **Nodular scleritis:** It presents with painful, tender, localized nodule and overlying episcleral inflammation. The scleral swelling is readily detectable with a fine beam of slit lamp moved over the affected area. Scleral nodule cannot be moved over the underlying tissues.
- **Necrotizing scleritis (with inflammation):** Extremely painful and presents with areas of avascularity in the sclera. Avascular areas may slough leading to scleral thinning, staphyloma formation and exposure of uveal tissues. It is associated with seropositive connective tissue disorders.
- **Scleromalacia perforans:** It is a painless necrotizing scleral inflammation usually seen in women with long-standing rheumatoid arthritis. Vessels of conjunctiva and episclera become extremely attenuated and episcleral tissue almost disappears. The condition presents without pain, minimal inflammation and change in color of sclera from white to yellow. The yellow areas disintegrate and get absorbed over a period of few weeks leaving the underlying choroid exposed.
- **Surgically induced necrotizing scleritis:** It is an immune mediated necrotizing scleritis that occurs following ocular surgery like cataract surgery, penetrating keratoplasty, muscle surgery, trabeculectomy or pterygium excision.

POSTERIOR SCLERITIS

Ocular Features

Symptoms: Blurred vision, pain, metamorphopsia

Signs: Shallow anterior chamber, disc swelling, serous retinal detachment, choroidal detachment, choroidal folds.

Investigations

FFA: Multiple areas of pin-point hyperfluorescence with pooling of the dye in the late phase

U/S: T-sign representing tenonitis, thickening of the posterior sclera

Associated Ocular Findings in Scleritis

1. **Keratitis:** Keratitis occurs in 50 percent of patients with scleritis. Sclerosing keratitis occurs adjacent to scleral inflammation. Deep stromal scarring may be seen. At times a central keratolysis with rapid tissue loss and perforation may occur typically in patients with rheumatologic disease.
2. **Iridocylitis** may be present in 50 percent patients with scleritis.
3. **Cataract** may occur secondary to inflammation or steroid therapy.
4. **Secondary glaucoma** may occur secondary to recurrent inflammation, steroid therapy or mechanical causes.
5. **Vitritis, macular edema, choroidal detachment, retinal detachment** may occur in posterior scleritis.

Systemic Associations

Connective tissue diseases—Rheumatoid arthritis, Wegener's granulomatosis, systemic lupus erythematosus, etc.

REFERENCES

1. Foster CS, Sainz de la Maza M. The Sclera, edited by Springer Verlag, 1994.
2. Paul J. Dubord, MD, Andrew Chalmers, MD, Scleritis and Episcleritis: Diagnosis and Management-Focal Points, American Academy of Ophthalmology Vol XIII; 9: Sep 1995;16:169-76.
3. Biswas J, Mittal S, Ganesh SK, Shetty NS, Gopal L. Posterior scleritis: Clinical profile and imaging characteristics: Ind J Ophthal 1998; 46: 195-202.
4. Jabs DA, Mudun A,. Dunn J. P and Marsh MJ. Episcleritis and Scleritis: Clinical Features and Treatment Results; Am J Ophthalmology 2000; 130:469-76.

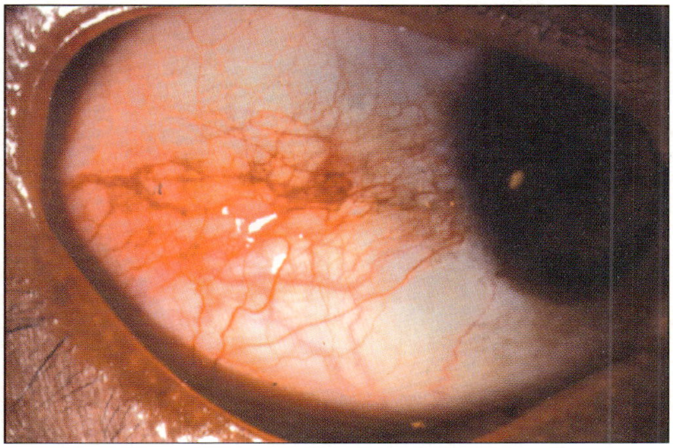

Fig. 29.1: Diffuse episcleritis which responded to topical non-steroidal anti-inflammatory drugs

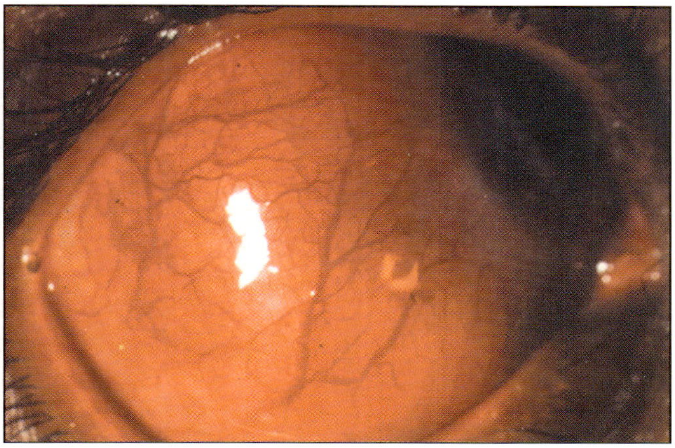

Fig. 29.2: Diffuse anterior scleritis in a 35-year-old lady who had recurrent attacks of redness since 2 year

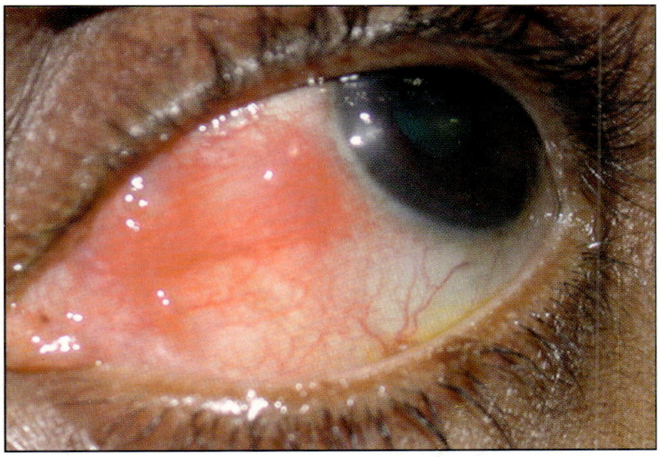

Fig. 29.3: Nodular anterior scleritis showing a tender scleral nodule

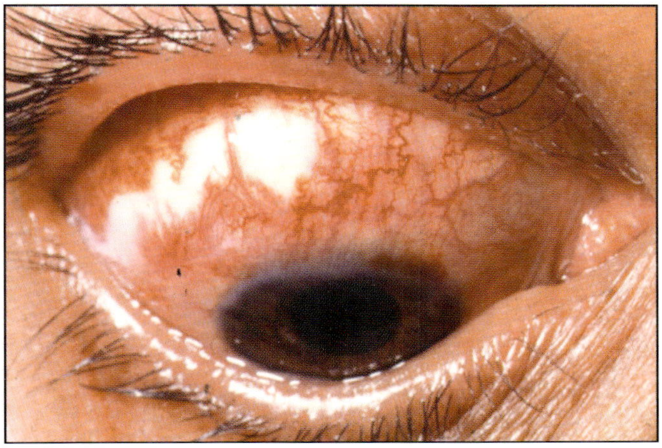

Fig. 29.4: Necrotizing anterior scleritis with an avascular patch in the superior sclera

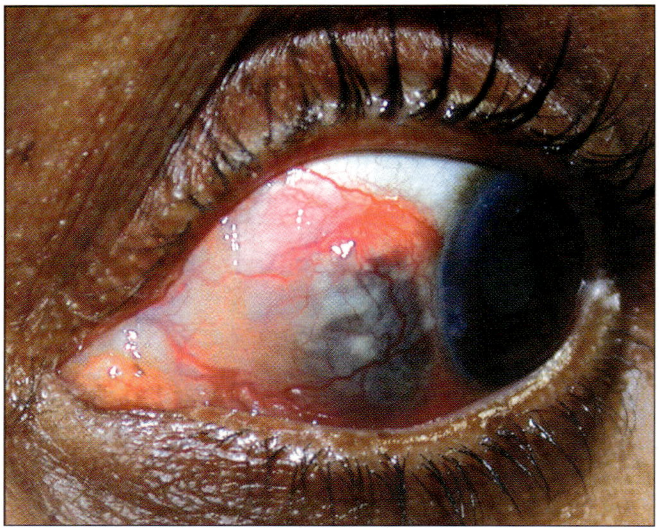

Fig. 29.5: Thinning of sclera with uveal tissue prolapse in advanced necrotizing scleritis

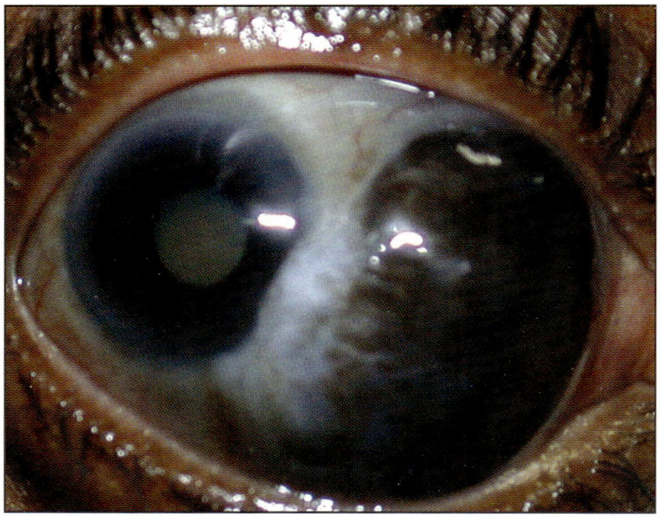

Fig. 29.6: Scleromalacia perforans in a 45-year-old lady suffering from severe rheumatoid arthritis

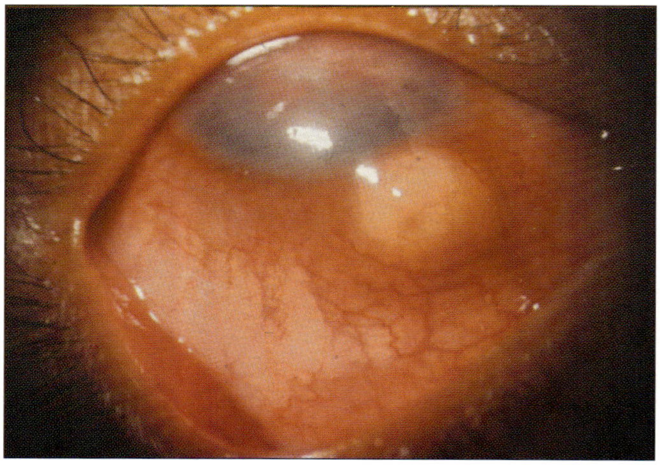

Fig. 29.7: Patch of scleritis diagnosed as infective scleritis

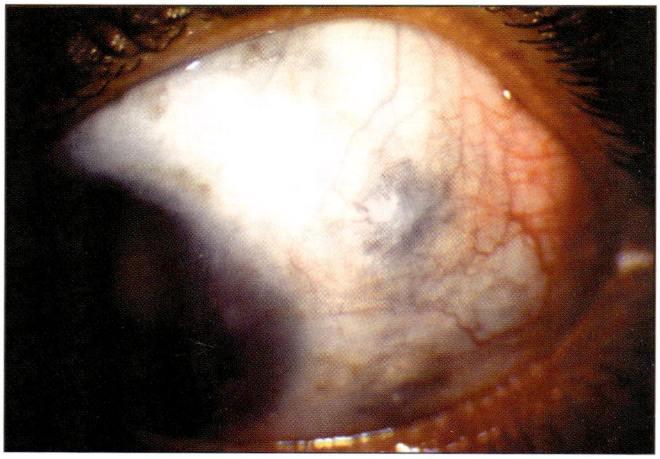

Fig. 29.8: Slit lamp photograph showing recurrent scleritis with a patch of thinned sclera

Posterior Scleritis

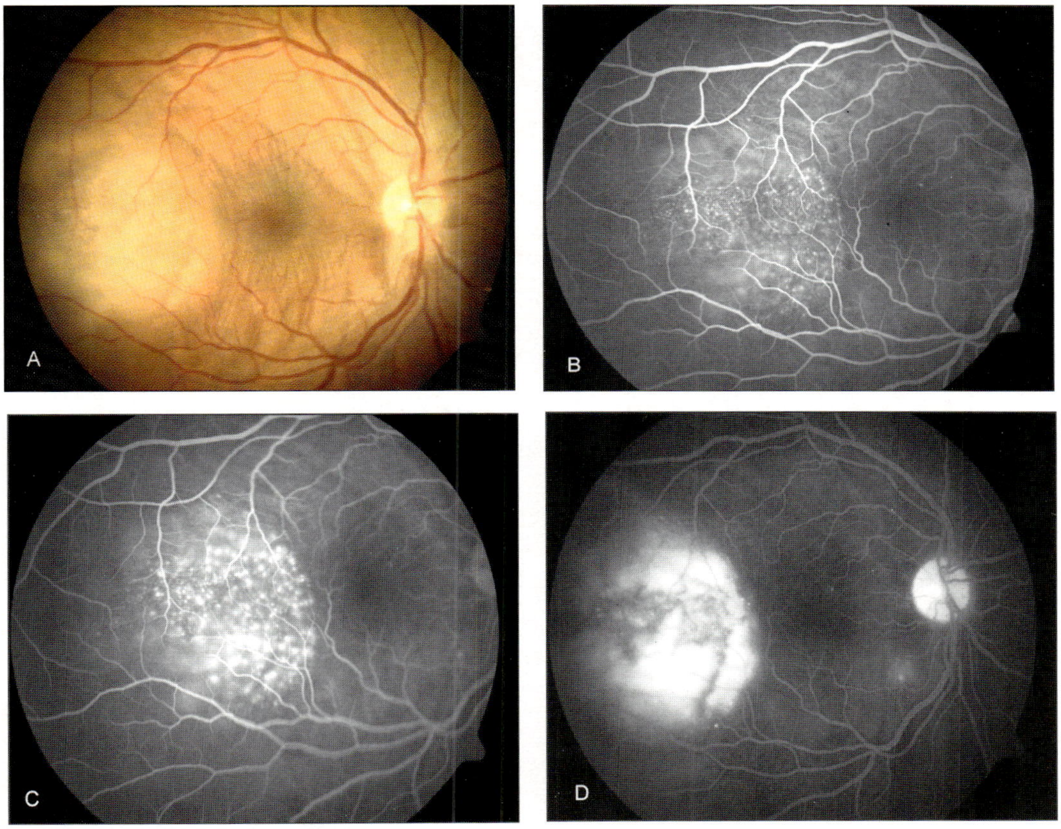

Figs 29.9A to D: A 45-year-old lady complained of sudden diminution of vision in right eye was diagnosed as posterior scleritis

A. Fundus photograph showed yellowish white elevated lesion temporal to macula along with choroidal folds
B. Fluorescein angiogram in the early phase showed pin-point hyperfluorescent leaks at the level of retinal pigment epithelium
C. Middle phase of the angiogram showed increase in the size and intensity of the hyperfluorescence
D. Late phase of the angiogram showed pooling of the dye in subretinal space

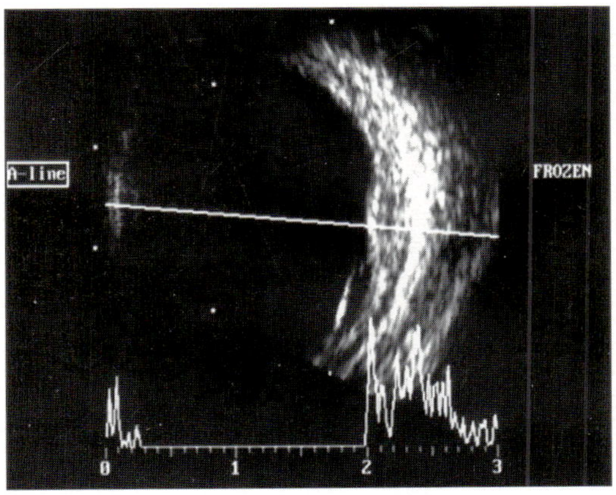

Fig. 29.10: Ultrasonography showing thickened posterior sclera and T-sign representing fluid in Tenon's capsule

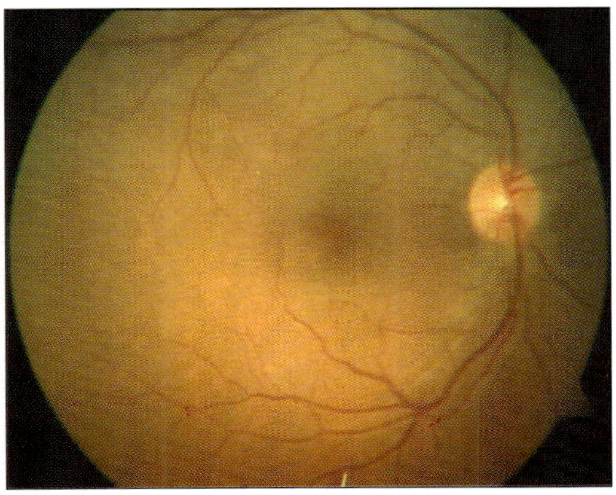

Fig. 29.11: Fundus photograph showing resolution of posterior scleritis following treatment with high-dose systemic steroids

INDEX